Pregnancy
Questions and Answers

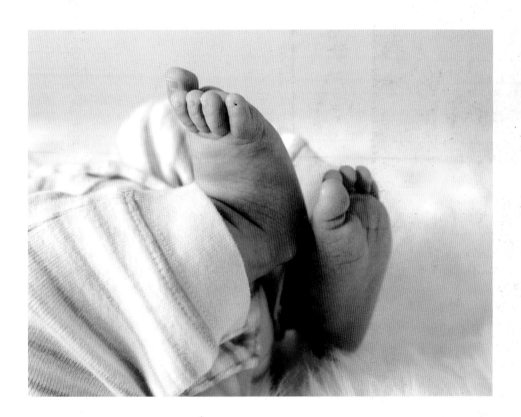

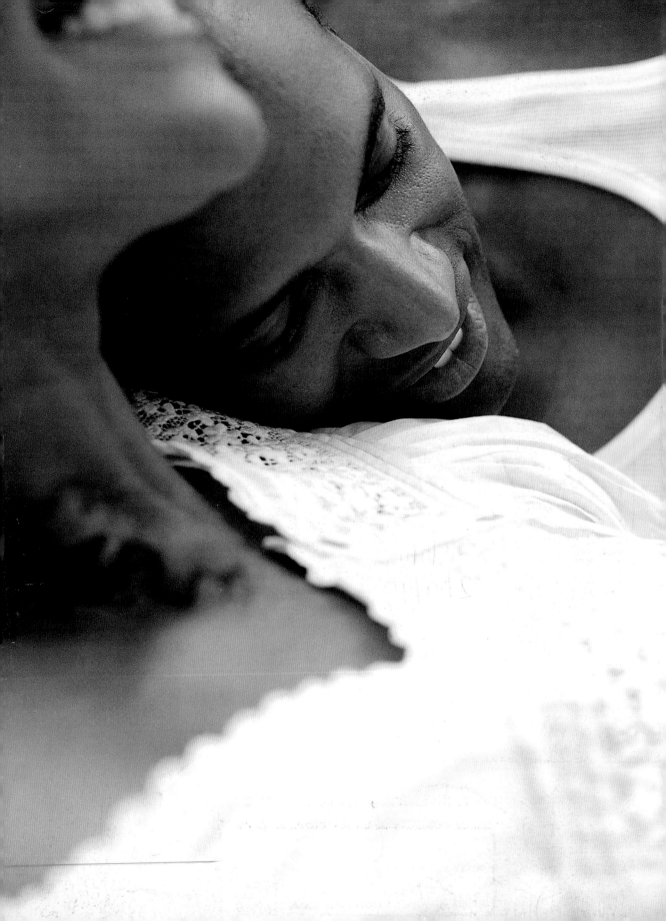

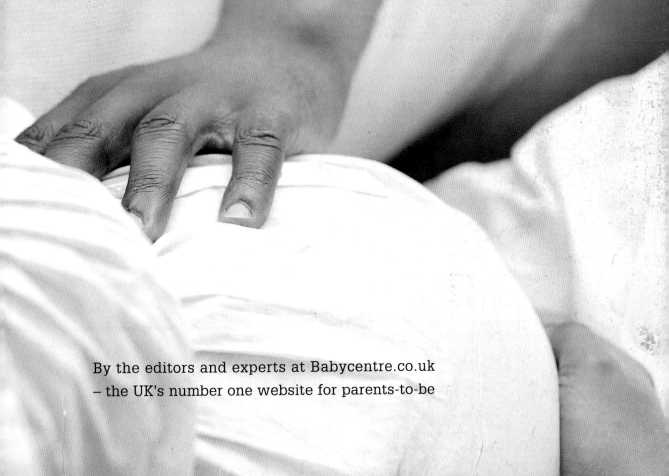
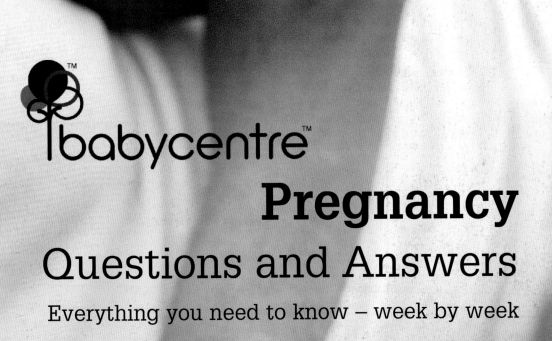

babycentre™

Pregnancy

Questions and Answers

Everything you need to know – week by week

By the editors and experts at Babycentre.co.uk
– the UK's number one website for parents-to-be

First published 2006 by Rodale

This paperback edition published 2009 by Rodale, an imprint of Pan Macmillan Ltd
Pan Macmillan, 20 New Wharf Road, London N1 9RR
Basingstoke and Oxford
Associated companies throughout the world
www.panmacmillan.com

Printed and bound in Italy by Printer Trento S.r.l.

1 3 5 7 9 8 6 4 2

A CIP record is available from the British Library

ISBN 978-1-9057-4435-0

Art direction and design Emma Forge
Compiling and editing Dawn Bates
Senior editor Liz Gough
Managing editor Miranda Smith
Photographer Vanessa Davies
Illustrator Mandy Miller
Picture researcher Davina Dunn
Design manager Jo Connor
DTP Keith Bambury, Sarah Pfitzner
Production manager Sara Granger

Notice

This book is intended as a reference volume only, not a medical manual. The information given
here is designed to help you to make informed decisions about your health. It is not intended as
a substitute for any treatment that may have been prescribed by your doctor. If you suspect that
you have a medical problem, we urge you to seek competent medical help. Mention of specific
companies, organizations or authorities in this book does not imply that they endorse the book.
Websites and telephone numbers were accurate at the time the book went to press.

Visit **www.panmacmillan.co.uk** to read more about all our books and to buy them. You will
also find features, author interviews and news of any author events, and you can sign up for
e-newsletters so that you're always first to hear about our new releases.

Foreword

You are thinking about getting pregnant, or you already know that you are going to have a baby (or babies!). You are at the beginning of a time in your life when your body, your emotions and your relationships will change dramatically – things will never be the same again. You and your partner will need to adjust and embrace the changes that will be required. Some women will feel happy, some anxious, some unhappy, about being pregnant. Many women feel all of these emotions. You are bound to have thousands of questions. Many of the books you will find to help you answer these questions are written by experts with the expert's own agenda in mind. This book is different. It is based on the questions that parents really ask. These questions are sent in by their hundreds to BabyCentre each week. The website has nearly 900,000 visitors each month, which means that BabyCentre is talking to, and listening to, huge numbers of women. This shows in this amazing book. The topics reflect the concerns of modern women and their partners. These are addressed with expertise coming from a number of professionals, but also from other women. Complex medical issues are tackled in ways that are easy to understand, based on good information, but are never simplistic. The book is also a goldmine of information on practical concerns, changing emotions, relationships, work, and sexuality and preparing to be a parent. While recognizing that some women will be single parents, Dad is never left out. The book is upbeat and modern with an easy layout and bright illustrations, but it never paints the over-romantic view of parenting and pregnancy and birth that leaves so many women and families feeling inadequate. It is very realistic. I wish this book had been around when I was pregnant. It is unique, thorough and helpful, and I recommend it as one of the most relevant, understanding and soundest sources of advice on pregnancy, birth and the early weeks of life.

Lesley Page PhD, MSc, BA, RM, RN

Joint Head of Midwifery and Nursing Women's Services at Guy's and St Thomas' NHS Foundation Trust and Visiting Professor of Midwifery Nightingale School of Nursing and Midwifery King's College London

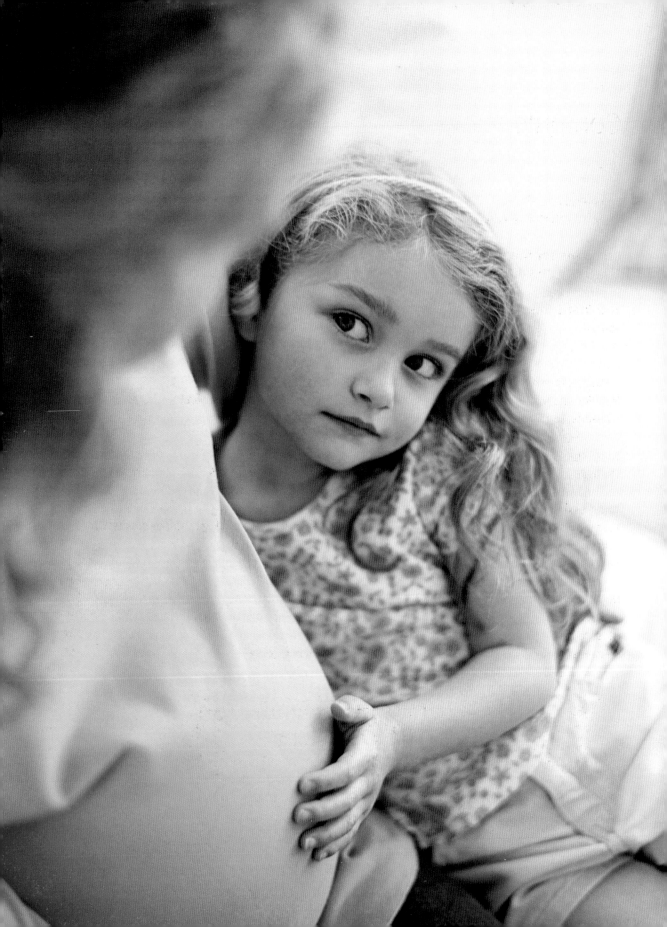

Contents

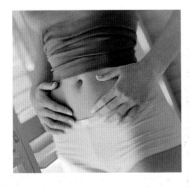
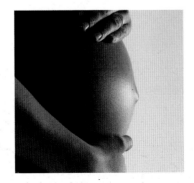
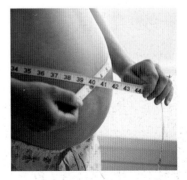

Introduction

Since we launched in 2000 we've seen BabyCentre thrive and grow to become the UK's leading online source of pregnancy and parenting information. That's because, at BabyCentre, we're dedicated to giving new, expecting and 'actively trying' parents the information, support and reassurance they need.

BabyCentre's articles and interactive tools are written and designed by a highly skilled, experienced team. We work with a medical advisory board and a team of experts to keep our content as fresh and up-to-date as possible. We also have a lively community of supportive parents and parents-to-be who are always there to offer a listening ear.

One of the most popular areas of BabyCentre is our Ask the Experts page. Each year, thousands of you email us with queries on everything from whether or not it's safe to eat cheese during pregnancy to how to encourage your baby to sleep more. It's our experts' answers to these questions that form the basis of this, our first-ever BabyCentre book. As well as answers to all the questions you've sent us over the years, you'll find fascinating facts and figures based on our onsite polls. Did you know, for example, that more than 80 per cent of you took longer to conceive than you expected? Or that 46 per cent of you crave sweet foods in pregnancy?

There are useful tips to help make your life easier and in-depth articles on important issues such as ultrasound scans and premature labour. At BabyCentre we believe that dads are just as important as their pregnant partners, so there's plenty for fathers-to-be to get their teeth stuck into as well.

We hope you enjoy reading *Pregnancy – Questions and Answers*. Whether you choose to dip in and out or use it as your pregnancy bible, you'll find it contains everything you need to know to keep you and your baby safe and healthy. People often say they are amazed at how well we understand the joys and concerns of parents and parents-to-be. We tell them it's very simple really: we're guided by the real experts – you!

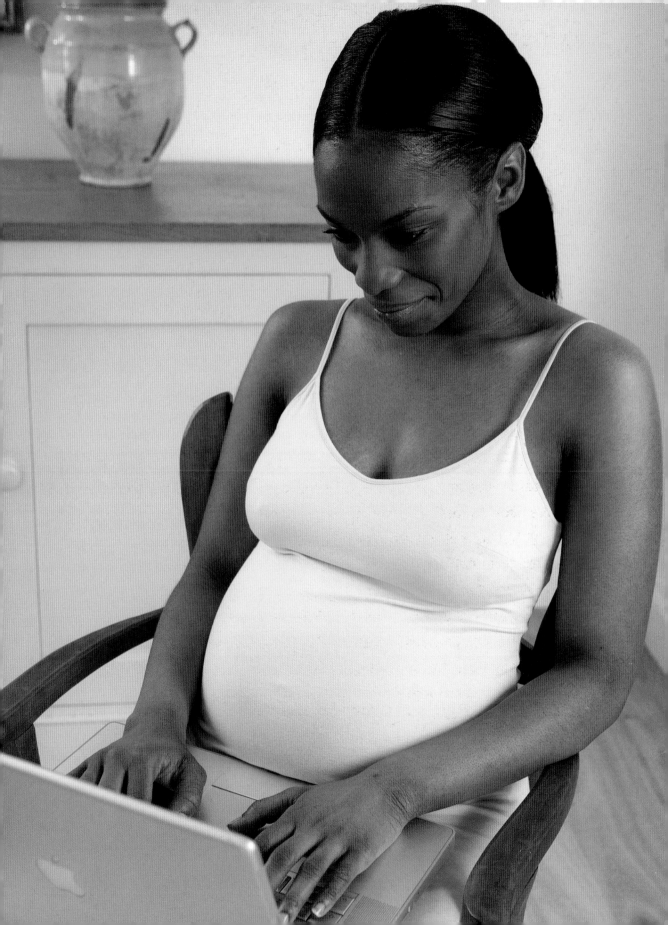

Meet the BabyCentre experts

It's the most amazing thing that's ever happened to you. It's also one of the scariest. Discovering you are pregnant for the first time brings up all sorts of emotions and lots of questions, too. But who do you turn to for advice and reassurance when your next midwife's appointment is still weeks away?

BabyCentre is there for you 24 hours a day from the very start. We pride ourselves on giving you the most accurate, up-to-date pregnancy, birth and parenting advice on the Net. All of our writers are experienced in writing for new and expectant parents – most of them are parents themselves. Many of them are drawn from our team of experts, which includes midwives, obstetricians, dieticians, physiotherapists, relationships experts and many more. And to make doubly sure you get only the most reliable information, all our medical articles are reviewed by a medical advisory board composed of leading experts in women's and children's health.

Whether you're still trying for a baby or you're already a new parent, our experts are there to guide you every step of the way. That's why thousands of you flock to BabyCentre.co.uk each month with queries on everything from how to get pregnant to breastfeeding and beyond. We read every single one of your emails and pass your queries on to our team of experts. Then we publish their answers on site so that other parents can stay fully informed, too.

Now there's a new way for you to benefit from the expertise we have gathered around us since we launched in 2000. In this attractive, easy-to-read book, you'll find answers to many of the queries you've sent us over the years. *Pregnancy – Questions and Answers* is based on real questions sent to us by real people. You'll find it gives you all the information you need from the moment you start trying for a baby right through to your new baby's first bath.

But enough from us – it's time to meet the BabyCentre experts.

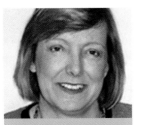

DAPHNE METLAND
**BABYCENTRE
EDITOR-IN-CHIEF**

*Daphne launched
BabyCentre in 2000. She
was formerly publishing
director for the NCT
and editor of* Parents
*magazine. She is co-
author of* Expecting:
Everything you need to
know about pregnancy
labour and birth, *and
is also an experienced
antenatal teacher.*

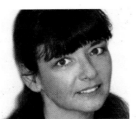

ANNA MCGRAIL
**BABYCENTRE
EXECUTIVE EDITOR**

*Anna McGrail has been
a writer and editor on
BabyCentre since 2000.
She is author of several
books including the
award-winning* You
and Your New Baby. *She
co-wrote, with Daphne
Metland,* Expecting:
Everything you need to
know about pregnancy,
labour and birth.

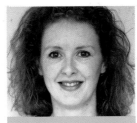

ALISON BOURNE
PHYSIOTHERAPIST

*Alison is a specialist
women's health
physiotherapist at
The Royal Hospital,
Chesterfield, where she
works with pregnant
women and new
mums. She also runs
antenatal and postnatal
exercise and advice
classes, and trains
other physiotherapists.*

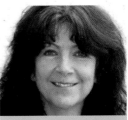

CHRISSIE
HAMMONDS
**MIDWIFE
SONOGRAPHER**

*Chrissie Hammonds
trained as a nurse and
midwife before gaining
a Master's degree in
medical ultrasound.
She is now a midwife
sonographer, university
lecturer and a member
of the UK National
Fetal Anomaly
Screening Group.*

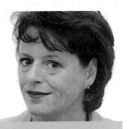

FIONA FORD
DIETICIAN

*Fiona Ford is a state
registered dietician and
has a Master's degree
in health research. She
works for the Centre
for Pregnancy Nutrition
at the University of
Sheffield. Among other
things, the Centre
hosts the national
Wellbeing Eating for
Pregnancy helpline.*

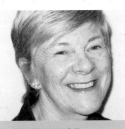

LESLEY PAGE
**PROFESSOR OF
MIDWIFERY**

*Professor Lesley
Page is Joint Head of
Midwifery and Nursing
Women's Services at
Guy's and St Thomas'
NHS Trust and a visiting
professor of midwifery
at King's College,
London. She is widely
published and has
lectured on midwifery
all over the world.*

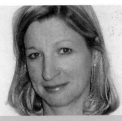

DR MAGGIE BLOTT
**CONSULTANT
OBSTETRICIAN**

*Dr Maggie Blott is a
consultant obstetrician
at the Royal Victoria
Infirmary in Newcastle-
upon-Tyne. She teaches
obstetrics and has a
particular interest in
maternal medicine
and labour ward
management. Her aim
is to support pregnant
women in their choices.*

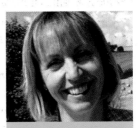

DR MORAG
MARTINDALE
GP

*Dr Morag Martindale
is a GP and family
planning doctor. She
was a contributing
author to the NCT
Book of Baby Care and
author of the NCT A-Z
of Child Health. She has
a particular interest
in women's health,
breastfeeding and
early parenting.*

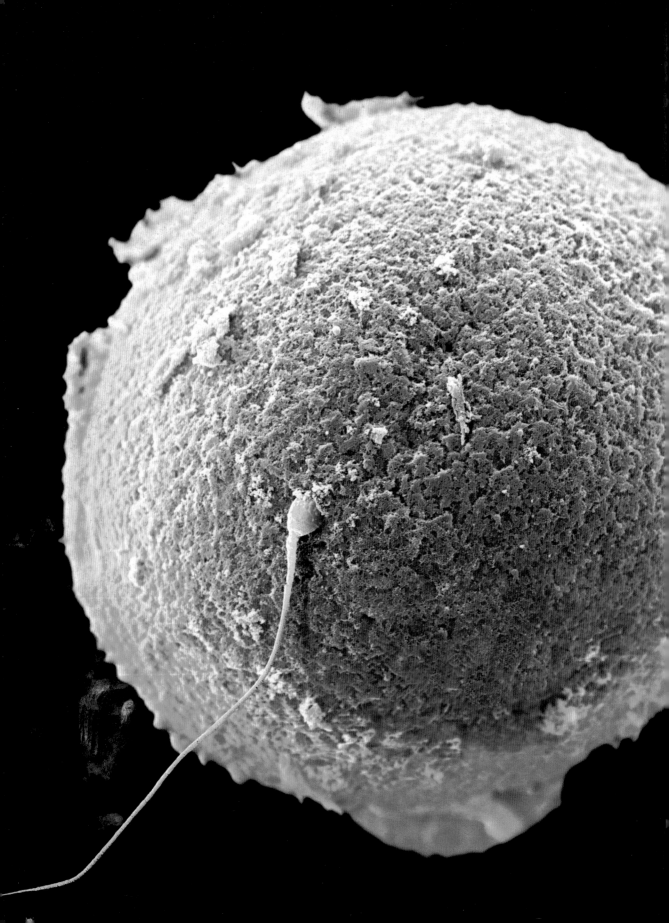

Preparing for **pregnancy**

Pregnancy is one of the biggest physical changes your body will ever undergo, so before you start trying for a baby it's advisable to make sure you're in good health – and the same goes for your partner. You can try to increase your likelihood of getting pregnant by learning to pinpoint exactly when you ovulate and by familiarizing yourself with the cycle of hormonal and physical changes that takes place in your body each month. However, ideally, try to stay relaxed and let nature take its course.

How can I get my body ready for pregnancy?

If you've made a decision to try for a baby, you and your partner should consider assessing your diet and lifestyle and make adjustments if necessary. If you start eating a healthier diet, cut back on alcohol and stop smoking now, you'll know that you're giving your baby-to-be the best start in life.

Should I attempt to lose my excess weight before I try for a baby?

It's beneficial to be close to your recommended weight, but consult your doctor before you embark on any diet or exercise plan. Any weight loss should be gradual – extreme weight loss from crash dieting may deplete your body's nutritional stores, which is far from ideal for pregnancy.

Do I need to improve my diet before I become pregnant?

It's a good idea to take stock of what you eat now. Getting into good habits before you conceive will promote good health for you and a healthy environment for your soon-to-be developing baby. As well as taking folic acid supplements (see right), you might want to ask yourself the following questions: Do I eat a balanced and varied diet that provides plenty of nutrients? Do I get at least 800 mg of calcium a day (the equivalent of three glasses of milk)? Do I suffer from heavy periods and, if so, is my iron intake adequate? Do I eat at least three meals per day? If you answered yes to all the questions, then your diet is fine. If you answered no, you'll need to make adjustments.

Should I cut back on alcohol?

If you drink alcohol regularly, you'll have to make adjustments. The current recommendations are to drink no more than one or two units of alcohol once or twice per week during pregnancy. A unit is ½ pt (¼ ltr) of standard strength beer, lager or cider, or a pub measure of a spirit. The average self-poured glass of wine is about two units.

Should I stop smoking?

Yes. On average, babies born to women who smoked during pregnancy are almost 226 g (½ lb) lighter than women who don't smoke. Low birthweight is one of the leading causes of infant illness, disability and death. The evidence that cigarette smoking may have other harmful effects is more controversial, but some other problems linked with smoking include ectopic pregnancy, miscarriage (see pp 18–19), problems with the placenta, vaginal bleeding and premature delivery.

Some studies have shown that smoking during pregnancy may harm the child's mental development and behaviour. Other research shows that certain birth defects may be more common in babies whose mother smoked during pregnancy.

QUICK TIP

In addition to taking folic acid, try to eat folate-rich foods such as dark green leafy vegetables (eg. spinach or kale), citrus fruits, nuts, whole grains, brown rice and fortified breads and cereals.

JUST FOR DAD

It's not just women who need to make dietary and lifestyle adjustments.

- **Vitamin C** *Eating plenty of foods rich in vitamin C reduces the risk of damaged sperm. A 227 ml (8 fl oz) glass of orange juice contains 124 mg of vitamin C. Aim for at least 60 mg daily, and more – at least 100 mg – if you smoke.*

- **Zinc** *Get more zinc in your diet: aim for at least 12–15 mg a day. Several studies show that even short-term zinc deficiencies can reduce semen volume and testosterone levels. Great sources include extra-lean minced beef and baked beans.*

- **Calcium and vitamin D** *You will need to increase your intake of calcium and vitamin D. Good sources of calcium include low-fat milk and yoghurt. There is vitamin D in milk and salmon.*

- **Alcohol** *Cut out or cut back on alcohol. While an occasional drink is generally considered safe, studies show that daily consumption of wine, beer or spirits can decrease testosterone levels and sperm count, and increase the number of abnormal sperm in semen.*

- **Drugs** *Do not take recreational drugs such as cannabis and cocaine, which can affect the brain chemistry responsible for releasing reproductive hormones. A father's drug use can also cause birth defects, while smoking cigarettes is known to affect sperm quality.*

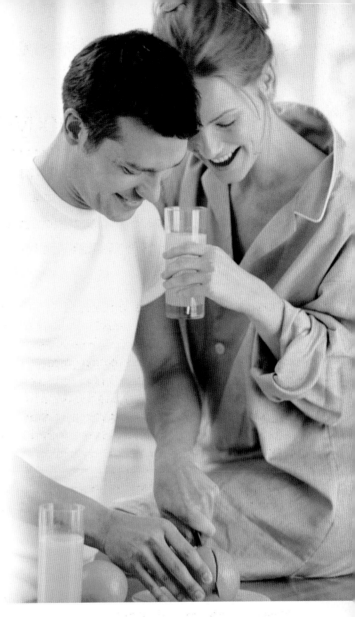

HEALTH KICK *For both men and women, foods and fertility are linked. If you and your partner stick to a balanced diet, you can boost your chances of conceiving and of having a healthy baby. Starting a health kick now will also stand you in good stead for pregnancy.*

Why do I need to take folic acid?

Folic acid reduces a baby's risk of having neural tube birth defects such as spina bifida. This is a serious congenital condition that occurs when the tube around the spinal cord fails to close completely. If you are trying to conceive (or at risk of becoming pregnant) take a folic acid supplement of 0.4 mg daily – also written as 400 micrograms (mcg). You should take this from the time you stop using contraception until at least the 12th week of pregnancy. Make sure that the supplement you use does not contain retinol (the animal form of vitamin A) or fish liver oil (see p 99). It is recommended that any woman who either has a neural tube defect, such as spina bifida, herself, or has had a child with a neural tube defect, or whose partner or immediate relative has a neural tube defect, takes a much higher dose of folic acid – 5 mg a day. This higher dose is also recommended for women who are taking anti-epileptic drugs, have coeliac disease (gluten intolerance) or have sickle cell disease.

How can I improve my chances of conceiving?

Relaxing and enjoying regular lovemaking is the best way to boost your chances of getting pregnant. However, if it's taking you and your partner a while to conceive, making sure you have sex around the time you ovulate may improve your chances – but try not to become too focused on timing your lovemaking.

What is ovulation?

Ovulation is when one or more eggs are released from one of your ovaries. This is the most fertile time of your menstrual cycle. Each month, 15 to 20 eggs mature inside the ovaries. The largest egg is expelled into the pelvic cavity and swept into the fallopian tube. Which ovary releases the egg is fairly arbitrary. Ovulation does not necessarily alternate between ovaries each cycle.

ASK THE EXPERT
DR MORAG MARTINDALE
GP

When should I stop taking my contraceptive pill if I want to get pregnant?

There are varied views on whether you should allow your body time to 'recover' from the effects of the pill before trying to get pregnant. Some experts recommend stopping the pill two to three months before trying to conceive because, as well as preventing you from ovulating, the pill causes changes in the lining of your uterus. If you did become pregnant, the embryo might not be able to embed itself in the uterine wall. The changes in the uterine lining take a few menstrual cycles to correct, so if you became pregnant immediately, you might have a higher risk of miscarriage. Some doctors recommend allowing your body to adjust to its natural cycle; others point out that the hormones from the pill are eliminated from your system as soon as you have your next period, so you should go ahead and try to conceive.

When should we have sex if I'm trying to conceive?

You are only fertile for a few days a month (around day 14 if you have a 28-day menstrual cycle). The egg released when you ovulate will survive no longer than 24 hours. However, because sperm can live for 72 hours you could still conceive if you've had sex 2–3 days before ovulation (see graph, right).

Don't become too focused on timing when you have intercourse. It can cause lovemaking to become a weary chore, undertaken when the date is right, even if neither you nor your partner are in the mood. Unfortunately, if you are not successful in conceiving, you may start to associate sex with the difficulty you are experiencing and this will cause further anxiety. If you are having sex without referring to the calendar every two or three days, then the sperm will be in the right place at the right time regardless of what your chart or predictor kit (see right) says.

Most couples actively trying for a baby will become pregnant within a year. If you have been trying for a year without success (or for six months if you're aged over 30), there may be a clinical reason why you're not conceiving and this can be investigated. Knowing this and allowing yourself to stop focusing on timing may bring some of the spontaneity and joy back into your sex life. Some experts actually think timing intercourse increases stress and, ironically, inhibits ovulation.

How can I tell when I'm most fertile?

As your menstrual cycle progresses, your cervical mucus increases in volume and changes texture, reflecting your body's rising levels of oestrogen. You are considered most fertile when the mucus becomes clear, slippery and stretchy. Many women compare mucus at this stage to raw egg whites. The role of mucus is to nourish, protect and speed the sperm on its way up through the uterus and into the fallopian tubes. About 20 per cent of women actually feel ovulatory activity, which can range from mild achiness to twinges of pain. Some women describe it as 'one-sided back ache' or a specific tenderness. The pain, called mittelschmerz, may last anywhere from a few minutes to a few hours. If you notice the same type of pain at roughly the same time each month, check the condition of your cervical mucus as well. Ovulatory pain can be a useful guide for some women.

Does a change in body temperature indicate that I'm ovulating?

Following ovulation, your temperature increases by 0.5 to 1.6 degrees. You won't feel the shift but you may be able to detect it by using a basal body temperature (BBT) thermometer. This temperature rise happens because releasing an egg stimulates the production of the hormone progesterone, which raises body temperature. You're most fertile in the two or three days before your temperature rises.

How do ovulation prediction kits work?

These kits detect the surge in luteinizing hormone (LH) just before ovulation (see graph, right). They can predict ovulation 24–36 hours in advance, but they're not foolproof because LH can surge with or without the release of an egg. False LH surges can

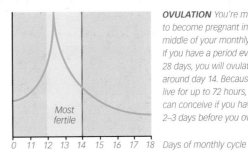

Most fertile

0 11 12 13 14 15 16 17 18   Days of monthly cycle

― Luteinizing hormone (LH)
― Ovulation

OVULATION *You're most likely to become pregnant in the middle of your monthly cycle. If you have a period every 28 days, you will ovulate on around day 14. Because sperm live for up to 72 hours, you can conceive if you have sex 2–3 days before you ovulate.*

also take place before the real one. For maximum accuracy, follow the kit's directions to the letter. If you have a 28-day cycle, start the test on day 11 and use it for six days (or however many days are recommended by the manufacturer). If your cycle is longer, say 35 days, start on day 14 for nine days. The women most likely to buy the kits – those with irregular cycles – may end up being the least satisfied with them. If your cycle is between 28–40 days, your ovulation range is between days 14 and 26. The kits provide five to nine days' worth of tests.

According to The Royal College of Obstetricians and Gynaecologists, however, there's no evidence that using LH detection methods or temperature checks (see left) to time intercourse improves outcome, and they discourage their use. In other words, studies show that the continued use of temperature checks and ovulation predictor kits does not improve your chances of getting pregnant in the long run. Charts can, however, provide other sorts of useful information about your monthly cycle and how regularly you ovulate.

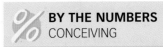

BY THE NUMBERS
CONCEIVING

Is it taking you much longer than you expected to conceive?

81% *Yes.*

19% *No.*

Source: Based on a BabyCentre.co.uk poll of 7,441 women.

Is there anything I can do to protect against having a miscarriage?

Miscarriage is the loss of a baby in the first 24 weeks of pregnancy. The majority are unexplained, although some lifestyle changes are thought to lower the risk. There is nothing that can be done to prevent a miscarriage once it's underway.

How common is miscarriage?

Sadly, it is very common. About 20 per cent of known pregnancies end in miscarriage and perhaps as many as three-quarters of all fertilized eggs are lost in the very early stages. About 98 per cent of women who miscarry do so in the first 13 weeks.

What causes a miscarriage?

Doctors aren't able to pinpoint the reason for most early miscarriages but it seems that a fetus that is abnormal in some way tends to miscarry.

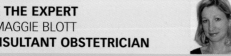

ASK THE EXPERT
DR MAGGIE BLOTT
CONSULTANT OBSTETRICIAN

What is an ectopic pregnancy and why does it happen?

This is a pregnancy that develops outside the uterus, usually in one of the fallopian tubes, but rare cases in the ovary or in the cervix have been known. An ectopic pregnancy most commonly occurs between the fourth and tenth week of pregnancy – usually from weeks five to seven. The most common reason is when the fallopian tube has been damaged, causing a blockage or narrowing that prevents the egg from reaching its destination. Instead, it implants in the wall of the tube. As the pregnancy grows, it causes pain and bleeding and, if not recognized, the tube can rupture, causing internal bleeding. This is a medical emergency.

At least half of all miscarriages in the first trimester of pregnancy are probably the result of chromosomal abnormalities that prevent the baby from developing normally. Later miscarriages – after 20 weeks – may be the result of an infection or an abnormality of the uterus or placenta. It can also happen if the cervix is not strong enough to keep the uterus closed until the baby is ready to be born.

What are the signs of a miscarriage?

The most obvious signs are period-like pains and heavy bleeding, which may include blood clots. However, you can miscarry without even knowing, especially in early pregnancy. Many women mistake a miscarriage for a late period. Some miscarriages are discovered only when the doctor or midwife cannot find the baby's heartbeat. This is known as a 'missed miscarriage', where the embryo has died but doesn't miscarry. Spotting (losing very small amounts of blood) is common in early pregnancy and may not be a problem, but always seek medical advice if you have any spotting or bleeding.

What can I do to reduce the risk of having a miscarriage?

If you smoke, giving up will reduce your risk of miscarriage, as will reducing your caffeine and alcohol intake. If you've had a miscarriage before, you may be advised to rest as much as possible for

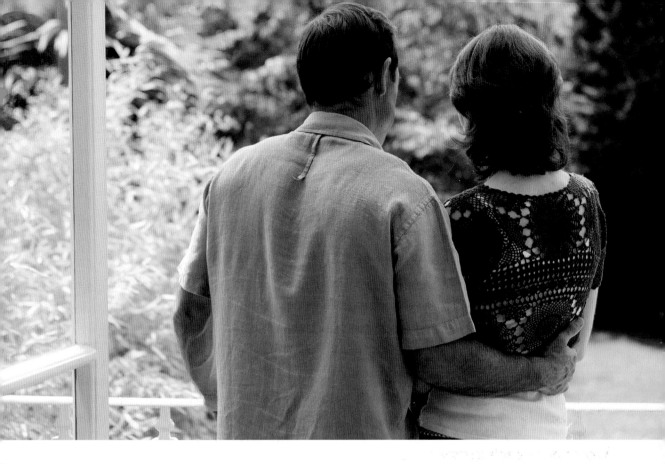

the first couple of months of pregnancy, although there's no actual evidence that this makes a difference. You might be advised to avoid sex until your pregnancy is well established. If you know that your cervix is weak because this was the reason for a previous miscarriage, you may be able to have a special stitch put round it to keep it closed.

Will a miscarriage affect my ability to conceive again?

No. Having a miscarriage does not mean that you have a fertility problem. Unless your doctor tells you otherwise, you will probably have a normal second pregnancy. Studies show that 50–75 per cent of women who have had three or more miscarriages go on to have healthy babies without medical treatment. After a first miscarriage, your chances of having another are no higher than before, and after two miscarriages, your risk of a third is only slightly increased. Give yourself time to recover physically and emotionally before you try to conceive again.

JUST THE FACTS
RISK FACTORS

The risk of miscarriage may be increased if you:

- *Smoke.*
- *Drink more than four cups of coffee a day or a lot of alcohol.*
- *Have had more than one miscarriage already.*
- *Have fibroids (non-cancerous tumours of the uterus) or an abnormally-shaped uterus.*
- *Have lupus.*
- *Have diabetes, kidney disease or thyroid disease, but the risk is lower if these are well managed.*
- *Have an infection, such as rubella, listeria or chlamydia, in early pregnancy .*
- *Are aged over 30. The miscarriage rate increases from age 30 and again from 35. Older women are more likely to conceive babies with chromosomal abnormalities and these pregnancies are more likely to be lost.*

How will I know if I'm pregnant?

Home pregnancy tests have made it easy for women to find out if they've conceived. Some come with two testing sticks so that you can double-check the result. It is also possible to go to your doctor's surgery for a pregnancy test. Some, but not all, women notice some physical signs and symptoms in the early weeks.

What are the signs of pregnancy?

If you're tuned in to your body's rhythms, you may begin to suspect you're pregnant soon after conception. But most women won't experience any symptoms until the fertilized egg attaches itself to the uterine wall several days after conception. Others may notice no signs for weeks. A missed period usually alerts most women to the possibility of pregnancy, and pregnancy tests can confirm a pregnancy within a few days of missing a period. Other early signs of pregnancy include a metallic taste in the mouth, very tender, sore breasts and a frequent need to pass urine. Nausea and sickness usually start at about six weeks and are worse from 8–10 weeks.

How does a home pregnancy test work?

A home pregnancy test measures the presence of the hormone human chorionic gonadotrophin (hCG) in your urine. This hormone is actually first secreted at the time the fertilized egg implants in the uterus (about six days after fertilization) by the cells that go on to form the placenta. Levels of the hormone build up rapidly in your body in the days following implantation. Usually, home pregnancy tests should be able to detect the hCG in your urine by the first day you miss your period. If you have a negative result when you first test, it may be because the levels of hCG have not yet reached a level where they can be detected so you may want to wait a few days then test again. Some tests are more sensitive – and consequently, more expensive – because they can detect pregnancy even if you have only a small amount of hCG in your system.

Are home pregnancy tests accurate?

If you follow directions to the letter, home pregnancy tests are 97 per cent accurate. But mistakes do happen, which is why some kits come with two tests. There are several reasons why a home pregnancy test may be negative: you may not be pregnant, or your body may not be making a normal amount of hCG (see above). If the test is negative but you still suspect you're pregnant, wait a few days and test again. False positives – when the test says you're pregnant but you're not – are rare.

Are home tests different from those performed by doctors?

Many clinics use home pregnancy tests to verify pregnancies. Occasionally, women are given blood tests. Both types of testing look for hCG, but a blood test is more sensitive and can determine whether you're pregnant just 6–8 days after you ovulate.

QUICK TIP

Perform a pregnancy test first thing in the morning when your urine is at its most concentrated.

WHAT'S YOUR DUE DATE?

To calculate your due date, find the first day of your last menstrual period (LMP) in bold. The date directly below it is your estimated date of delivery (EDD). If your last period started on January 11, for instance, then your EDD is October 18. Be aware, though, that a normal, full-term baby can arrive at any time between three weeks before and two weeks after your due date.

January 1 2 3 4 5 6 7 8 9 10 11 12 13 14 15 16 17 18 19 20 21 22 23 24 25 26 27 28 29 30 31
Oct/Nov 8 9 10 11 12 13 14 15 16 17 18 19 20 21 22 23 24 25 26 27 28 29 30 31 1 2 3 4 5 6 7

February 1 2 3 4 5 6 7 8 9 10 11 12 13 14 15 16 17 18 19 20 21 22 23 24 25 26 27 28
Nov/Dec 8 9 10 11 12 13 14 15 16 17 18 19 20 21 22 23 24 25 26 27 28 29 30 1 2 3 4 5

March 1 2 3 4 5 6 7 8 9 10 11 12 13 14 15 16 17 18 19 20 21 22 23 24 25 26 27 28 29 30 31
Dec/Jan 6 7 8 9 10 11 12 13 14 15 16 17 18 19 20 21 22 23 24 25 26 27 28 29 30 31 1 2 3 4 5

April 1 2 3 4 5 6 7 8 9 10 11 12 13 14 15 16 17 18 19 20 21 22 23 24 25 26 27 28 29 30
Jan/Feb 6 7 8 9 10 11 12 13 14 15 16 17 18 19 20 21 22 23 24 25 26 27 28 29 30 31 1 2 3 4

May 1 2 3 4 5 6 7 8 9 10 11 12 13 14 15 16 17 18 19 20 21 22 23 24 25 26 27 28 29 30 31
Feb/Mar 5 6 7 8 9 10 11 12 13 14 15 16 17 18 19 20 21 22 23 24 25 26 27 28 1 2 3 4 5 6 7

June 1 2 3 4 5 6 7 8 9 10 11 12 13 14 15 16 17 18 19 20 21 22 23 24 25 26 27 28 29 30
Mar/Apr 8 9 10 11 12 13 14 15 16 17 18 19 20 21 22 23 24 25 26 27 28 29 30 31 1 2 3 4 5 6

July 1 2 3 4 5 6 7 8 9 10 11 12 13 14 15 16 17 18 19 20 21 22 23 24 25 26 27 28 29 30 31
Apr/May 7 8 9 10 11 12 13 14 15 16 17 18 19 20 21 22 23 24 25 26 27 28 29 30 1 2 3 4 5 6 7

August 1 2 3 4 5 6 7 8 9 10 11 12 13 14 15 16 17 18 19 20 21 22 23 24 25 26 27 28 29 30 31
May/June 8 9 10 11 12 13 14 15 16 17 18 19 20 21 22 23 24 25 26 27 28 29 30 31 1 2 3 4 5 6 7

September 1 2 3 4 5 6 7 8 9 10 11 12 13 14 15 16 17 18 19 20 21 22 23 24 25 26 27 28 29 30
June/July 8 9 10 11 12 13 14 15 16 17 18 19 20 21 22 23 24 25 26 27 28 29 30 1 2 3 4 5 6 7

October 1 2 3 4 5 6 7 8 9 10 11 12 13 14 15 16 17 18 19 20 21 22 23 24 25 26 27 28 29 30 31
July/Aug 8 9 10 11 12 13 14 15 16 17 18 19 20 21 22 23 24 25 26 27 28 29 30 31 1 2 3 4 5 6 7

November 1 2 3 4 5 6 7 8 9 10 11 12 13 14 15 16 17 18 19 20 21 22 23 24 25 26 27 28 29 30
Aug/Sept 8 9 10 11 12 13 14 15 16 17 18 19 20 21 22 23 24 25 26 27 28 29 30 31 1 2 3 4 5 6

December 1 2 3 4 5 6 7 8 9 10 11 12 13 14 15 16 17 18 19 20 21 22 23 24 25 26 27 28 29 30 31
Sept/Oct 7 8 9 10 11 12 13 14 15 16 17 18 19 20 21 22 23 24 25 26 27 28 29 30 1 2 3 4 5 6 7

Will having irregular periods affect when I can do a pregnancy test?

If you have an irregular monthly cycle, it may be harder to work out if you're pregnant. You might just have a late period again, or you may have actually conceived. Allow for your longest menstrual cycle in recent months before doing a pregnancy test. If you have recently stopped taking the contraceptive pill (see p 16), you may not know how long your natural cycle is so you may end up testing too soon. If your test is negative in these situations, you should do another pregnancy test in three days if your period hasn't started.

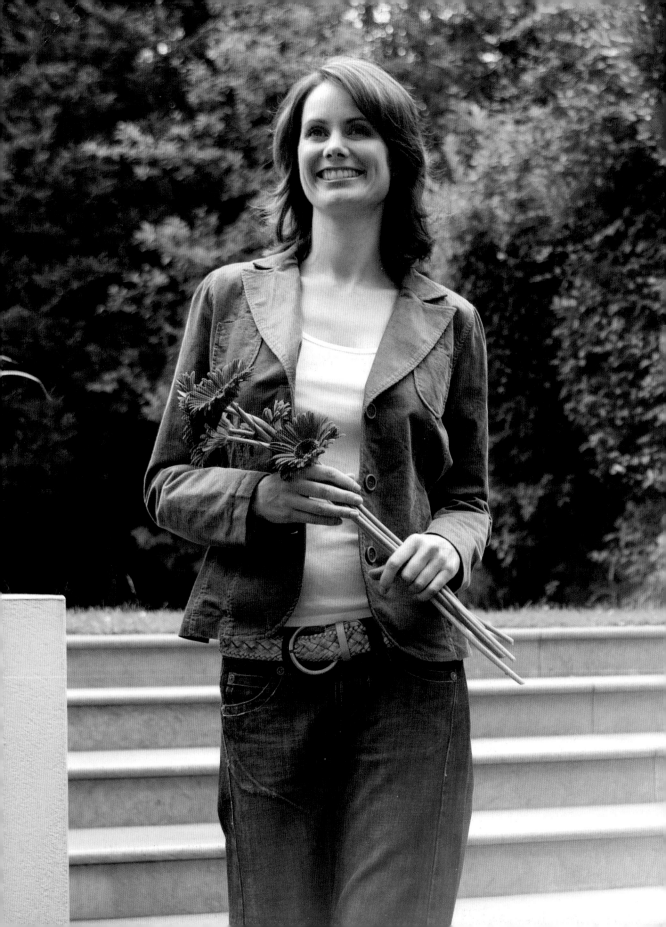

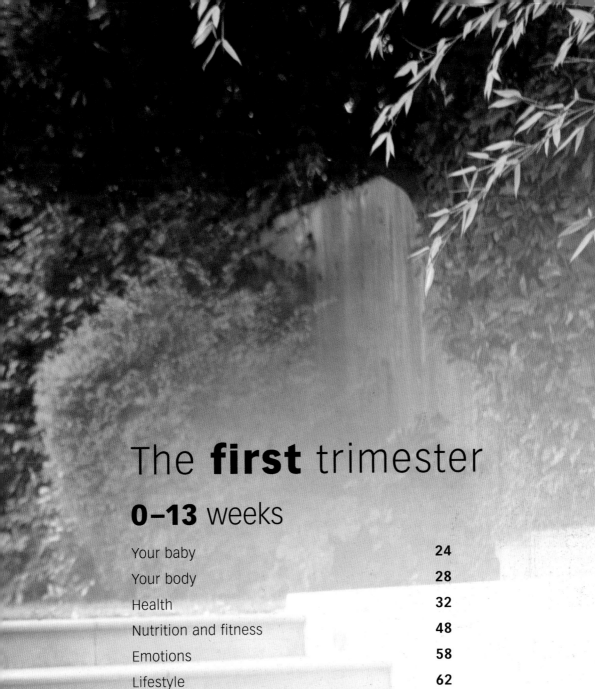

The **first** trimester

0–13 weeks

Congratulations – you're pregnant! In the next three months, an amazing number of changes will take place in your body and in your life. You no doubt have lots of questions – about the antenatal care you'll receive, the tests you'll be offered, what symptoms to expect and how to handle them, and whether to break the news to family and friends. Fear not! In this section you'll find all the answers and reassurance you need.

0–13 weeks How will my baby develop?

Fetal development in the first 13 weeks of pregnancy is rapid. Once the egg has been fertilized in week three, it divides and multiplies to produce a cluster of cells that will, by the end of this trimester, have been gradually transformed into a tiny human being that has eyes, ears, fingers and toes.

Your baby at six weeks

The embryo has nestled into the soft lining of your uterus and will derive its nourishment from the yolk sac. This churns out red blood cells and helps to nourish your baby until your placenta starts functioning at around week 12. The next few weeks are the time when your baby is most vulnerable to anything that might interfere with his development – and the time when you need to be most careful about anything that might harm him. Also present are the amniotic sac that surrounds your baby and the amniotic fluid that cushions him.

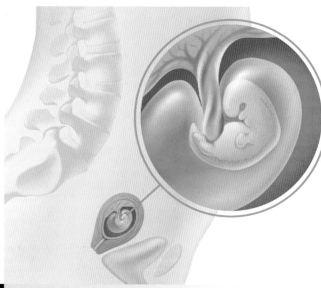

From embryo to fetus

At six weeks, the embryo measures approximately 1.5 cm (0.5 in) in length and has paddle-like limbs. The lenses of the eyes appear at around six weeks. The embryo floats in an amniotic sac, attached to what will become the developing placenta by an umbilical cord (centre left). Nutrients and oxygen pass from the mother to her embryo through the umbilical cord, while waste products travel in the opposite direction. By nine weeks, the embryo will be called a fetus.

Weeks 0–2

Your doctor or midwife will calculate the start of your pregnancy from the first day of your last menstrual period (LMP), but you are not actually pregnant in the first two weeks. The start of your pregnancy is the point at which you ovulate and the egg is fertilized, around the 14th day of an average monthly cycle. The actual pregnancy then lasts around 38 weeks from conception to birth.

Weeks 3–4

Just after ovulation a momentous meeting takes place. A microscopic sperm cell breaks through the protective barrier surrounding your egg and fertilizes it. A baby is in the making. Over the next day or so, your DNA will combine with your partner's DNA within the fertilized egg. Genetic material from each is being merged into the blueprint for your baby-to-be.

Throughout this process, the fertilized egg that is travelling down your fallopian tube towards your uterus is dividing and multiplying into a ball of 16 identical cells. This is known as a blastocyst. By the time the egg reaches your uterus three or four days later, and begins burrowing into the lining there a day or two after that, the ball of cells will be stretched like a double-layered water balloon.

The outer layer of this ball of cells will eventually form the placenta, the organ that delivers life-sustaining oxygen and nutrients to your baby throughout pregnancy; the inner layer will become your baby; and the fluid-filled centre will become the amniotic sac that cushions him as he grows.

Week 5

The ball of cells dividing in your uterus is now an embryo, about the size of an apple pip. What will become amniotic fluid begins to collect and in the weeks and months ahead, this fluid will cushion your developing baby. Nerve growth begins when a sheet of cells on the back of the embryo folds in the middle to form a tube. This is called the neural tube – from which the brain, backbone, and spinal cord and nerves will sprout. The top layer will also give rise to your baby's skin, hair, nails, mammary and sweat glands. At one end, the tube enlarges to form the brain's major sections. Folic acid (see p 15) is essential to the healthy formation of this neural tube, which is why women are advised to take folic acid supplements while they're trying to conceive and in early pregnancy.

In fact, the next five weeks are especially critical to your baby's development. The heart and the circulatory system begin to appear. The heart, which is no bigger than a poppy seed, begins to beat. The lungs, intestines and the urinary system also start to develop at around this time.

In the meantime, the early version of the placenta, the chorionic villi, and the umbilical cord which delivers nourishment and oxygen to your baby, are already working.

Week 6

At this point, however, the embryo still looks more like a tadpole than a human. Major organs, such as the kidneys, have begun to develop, and the neural tube, which connects the brain and spinal cord, closes.

The embryo's upper and lower limb buds begin to sprout – these will form your baby's arms and legs. The intestines are developing inside the umbilical cord and the appendix is already in place.

Below the opening that will later be your baby's mouth, small folds exist where the neck and the lower jaw will eventually develop. As early as this week, facial features are already appearing. Nostrils are becoming distinct and the earliest version of the retinas in the eyes are forming.

JUST THE FACTS
YOUR BABY'S FIRST TRIMESTER HIGHLIGHTS

During this trimester, your baby will:
- *Start out the size of an apple pip and grow to be the size of a king-size prawn.*
- *Form all the necessary organs and body parts, including the heart and the eyes.*
- *Start to move, but you won't be able to feel this until well into the second trimester.*
- *Be most vulnerable during weeks 4–10, so try to take extra care of yourself at this time.*

Your baby at week 12

Your baby's head is disproportionately large in relation to his body; his forehead bulges with his developing brain, and his eyes are sealed shut. There's no question that his appearance is already distinctly human. His eyes have moved to the front of his head, and his ears are in the right position. His fingers will soon begin to open and close, his toes will curl, his eye muscles will clench and his mouth will make sucking movements. Around this time, if you were to prod your abdomen, he would squirm in response, though you won't feel it.

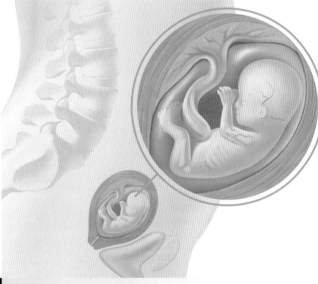

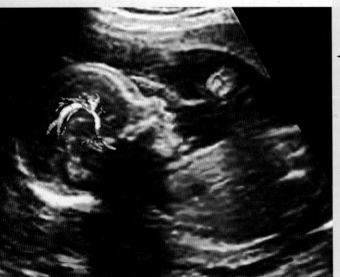

Brain development

As the fetus develops, fetal nerve cells multiply rapidly and synapses (neurological connections in the brain) begin to form. This coloured doppler ultrasound scan shows the blood vessels in the brain of a healthy 12-week-old fetus. Doppler ultrasound uses high-frequency sound to detect whether fetal development is normal. The technique is also able to detect movement, such as blood flow, and shows the flow of fluids in different directions as different colours.

Week 7

By this week the embryo is about the size of a small bean. The heart has already divided into the right and left chambers and is beating about 150 times a minute – roughly twice the rate of an adult heart. Fingers and toes start to develop. Around this stage of pregnancy, your baby begins to make his first movements, but you won't feel them for some time yet.

Week 8

In theory your baby is still an embryo because he has the remains of a small tail, which will become the coccyx or 'tailbone'. The heart and brain are becoming more complex, the eyelid folds are forming, the tip of the nose is present, and the arms now bend at the elbows and curve slightly. The teeth and palate are forming, while the ears continue to develop. Your baby's skin is paper thin, making his veins visible.

Week 9

This is the critical stage when your baby's organs are forming. He is now quite active – constantly moving and shifting. His arms have grown and his hands are now flexed at the wrists and meet over the heart. His legs are lengthening and his feet may be long enough to meet in front of the body.

Week 10

So many changes have taken place that your baby has stopped being an embryo and is now officially called a fetus. Your baby weighs under 10 g (a fraction of an ounce) but is poised for rapid growth. All the body parts are present, including arms, legs, eyes and other organs, though they're not yet fully formed. The sex of the fetus can't be identified by ultrasound yet, but the genitals have begun to form. By now the placenta is able to support most of the critical job of producing hormones.

Week 11

Your baby will double in size in the next three weeks. He is now swallowing and kicking, and all the major organs are fully developed. More minute details are appearing too, like fingernails and hair. The external sex organs are beginning to show and, in a few weeks, will be developed enough to tell whether you're going to have a boy or a girl. His intestines, which started out as a large swelling in the umbilical cord, will begin moving into the abdominal cavity about now.

Week 12

Your baby is now fully formed, and has all his tiny body parts from toothbuds to toenails. He measures about 6 cm (2.5 in), roughly the length of your thumb. His fingers and toes have separated and some of his bones are beginning to harden. He is busy kicking and stretching; his movements are so fluid they look like water ballet. His fingers and toes have fully separated and his face is changing. The eyes, which started out on the sides of his head, have moved closer together and his ears are almost in their final position.

Week 13

This is when the tissues and organs that have already formed in your baby's body rapidly grow and mature. Your baby has acquired more reflexes and will now move if you press your abdomen: touching his palms will make his fingers close, touching the soles of his feet will make his toes curl down and touching his eyelids will make his eye muscles clench.

0–13 weeks How will my body change this trimester?

The challenge in the first three months is coping with pregnancy symptoms brought on by hormonal changes. These symptoms should ease as the placenta takes over hormone production and you may start to see the first signs of your 'bump'.

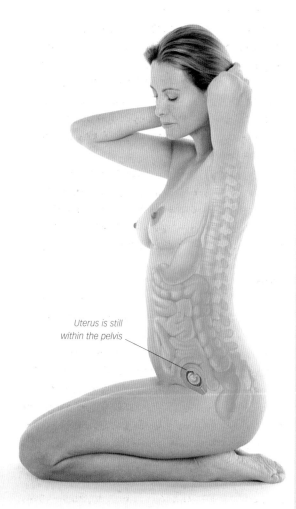

Uterus is still within the pelvis

YOUR UTERUS *You may not look or even feel pregnant, but your uterus is expanding to accommodate your growing baby. Before you became pregnant, your uterus was the size of a clenched fist; now it's as big as a grapefruit. As it grows you may feel some abdominal cramping and mild twinges.*

Your body at 6 weeks

Like most women, you are likely to feel pregnant long before you look pregnant because of the hormonal changes that are taking place in your body. Hormone levels rise dramatically in the early weeks of pregnancy. Oestrogen levels increase to stimulate the development of milk glands that will enable you to breastfeed your baby but, in turn, cause your breasts to feel sore and sensitive (see pp 40–41). Progesterone levels increase to maintain your pregnancy, but also lead to unwanted early pregnancy symptoms such as fatigue (see pp 42–3) and morning sickness (see below and pp 44–5). Thankfully your body will have adapted to these hormonal changes by the second trimester.

Morning sickness

Three out of four pregnant women suffer from nausea – and sometimes vomiting – especially in the first trimester. For many, the symptoms are worse in the morning, hence the name. For others, stomach churning lasts morning, noon and night. Queasiness usually begins at around week 6 and has passed by around week 14. It is most likely caused by pregnancy hormones, although doctors still aren't sure why and how it happens.

Weeks 0–2

Doctors calculate the start of your pregnancy from the first day of your last period, so you are not actually pregnant in the first two weeks. Hormones in the first two weeks of the cycle prepare your body for a possible pregnancy, thickening the lining of the uterus ready for a fertilized egg.

Week 3

Though many will try, only one of the awaiting army of sperm will successfully fertilize your egg. After its trip down your fallopian tube is complete, the fertilized egg nestles into your womb and sets up residence for the next nine months or so. You won't know that you've conceived, but you may soon start to notice the early signs of pregnancy: fatigue, frequent urination, and tender, swollen breasts. You may also have a little spotting for a few days around the time your period is due. Some women confuse this implantation bleeding with menstruation, but not all women experience it.

Week 4

Now that 28 days have passed since you last menstruated, the period that you've been expecting may be a no-show. If so, a home pregnancy test (see p 20) may be able to confirm your news. You might also want to start taking folic acid (see p 15) if you're not already taking it. Seek advice from your doctor if you are on any medication; the next few weeks are critical to your baby's development and some drugs will not be safe now.

Week 5

If you are used to regular exercise, it is safe to continue in pregnancy until a time when your bump gets in the way, making some forms of exercise more difficult. If you are not used to exercising, then, strange as it may seem, this is a good time to start. Exercise helps you develop good muscle tone, strength and endurance. It helps you manage the extra weight you'll put on (or prevent you putting on too much more), gets you fit for labour – and makes getting your figure back after birth easier too.

Week 6

Pregnancy symptoms continue or start this week. Many women notice nausea that can last all day (see pp 44–5), fatigue (see pp 42–3), the discomfort of sore breasts (see pp 40–41) and a need to urinate more often. All are normal, all are annoying, but the good thing is that they're simply a part of being pregnant and they won't last forever. Some women also get headaches.

It's important to eat well at every stage of pregnancy (see pp 48–9) so that your baby gets all the nutrients he needs (see pp 52–3). Small, regular meals and plenty of drinks can help to prevent indigestion and combat nausea and fatigue.

Week 7

The outside world won't yet see any sign of the dramatic developments taking place inside you, but tiredness and nausea can make you feel low, especially as you try to cope at work (see pp 68–9). To compensate, offload as much as you can at home and involve your partner in your pregnancy at the same time. Put yourself first and try to prioritize rest. You may have thought that disturbed nights start when the baby has arrived, but many women find their sleep is disrupted from the beginning of pregnancy. Sometimes the cause is physical – your growing uterus puts pressure on your bladder necessitating trips to the toilet during the night. Or perhaps sore breasts (see pp 40–41) are preventing you from getting comfortable.

JUST THE FACTS
YOUR FIRST TRIMESTER HIGHLIGHTS

During this trimester, you will:

- Most likely experience nausea, fatigue, sore breasts and frequent urination.
- Gain about 2.25 g (5 lb) in weight.
- Experience a range of different emotions.
- Notice your breasts increasing in size and changing in appearance.
- Go for your booking appointment (see p 32) and possibly have a nuchal translucency scan (see p 36).

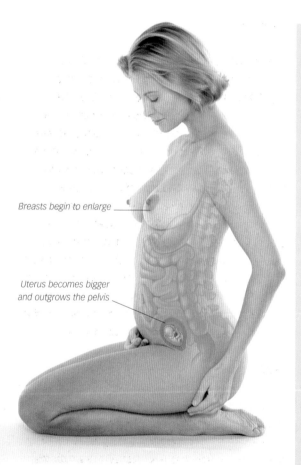

Breasts begin to enlarge

Uterus becomes bigger and outgrows the pelvis

***BEGINNING TO SHOW** Although you have probably felt pregnant for many weeks, the physical changes will only have been slight up to now. By week 12, however, your stomach will have begun to swell and your waist will have thickened. Your breasts will have enlarged slightly and the nipples may be darker. Your weight gain may depend on how much morning sickness you've suffered – some women actually lose weight because of nausea, but this won't harm your baby.*

Your body at 12 weeks

By this week of pregnancy your uterus will be almost big enough to fill your pelvis. You might even be able to feel the top of your uterus – called the fundus – above the middle of your pubic bone. As it continues to increase in size, the uterus will gradually outgrow the confines of your pelvis and begin to rise into your abdominal cavity. This is when your 'bump' will begin to appear, and hiding your pregnancy may start to become more difficult.

Your body will begin to adjust to your changing hormone levels about now, which should mean that morning sickness and those rollercoaster emotions become a thing of the past.

Cramps

You may feel faint abdominal cramps or a stretching sensation early in your pregnancy. As long as it's mild and short-lived, it is perfectly normal and nothing to be alarmed about. It's usually caused by your growing uterus and the stretching of the abdominal ligaments to accommodate it. Always call your doctor or midwife if you have persistent, severe cramps or abdominal pain with or without accompanying symptoms.

Week 8

In early pregnancy many women feel as if they are on an emotional rollercoaster (see pp 58–9) – ecstatic to be pregnant one moment only to be in tears at the prospect of parenthood the next. The slightest things may set you off. You'll be reassured to know that it's common to have mood swings at this stage and that they are caused by hormonal changes. These surging hormones and pregnancy anxieties can also result in vivid dreams.

Week 9

You're unlikely to have gained much weight, but your breasts will have grown. Your blood volume will have begun to increase; by the end of pregnancy, you'll have 40–50 per cent more blood to meet your baby's demands. The extra demands on your circulation make you prone to varicose veins (see p 137) and piles (see p 145).

Week 10

Physically you're unlikely to look pregnant unless this isn't your first pregnancy, but you may feel very tired (see pp 42–3) and sick (see pp 44–5) – not necessarily in the mornings – so cosset yourself. Pregnancy hormones can also play havoc in other ways. Many women suffer from headaches and, unfortunately, these hormones also help make the perfect environment for vaginal thrush.

Week 11

You're nearing the end of the first three months of pregnancy – your first trimester – and your uterus is now almost big enough to fill your pelvis. Though you probably won't need to go up a dress size for several more weeks yet, you may notice that your waist is thickening. Make sure you're drinking plenty: try to drink eight glasses of liquid every day – limiting caffeinated drinks (see p 51). Do not drink too much before bedtime to reduce the likelihood of you having to get up to go to the toilet during the night. If your sleep is disturbed for other reasons, such as anxiety or physical discomforts, then you may be tempted to take a remedy but medication shouldn't be your first course of action during pregnancy.

Week 12

You should have had your first antenatal check-up with a midwife, generally known as the booking appointment (see p 32), by now. This is when your midwife makes arrangements for your care throughout your pregnancy and in the weeks after the birth. She will also take some blood and urine tests and ask you questions about your medical history and lifestyle, and that of your partner.

One of the most exciting parts of antenatal visits is hearing your baby's rapid heartbeat magnified by the Sonicaid listening device many midwives use. Don't be alarmed if your midwife cannot find a heartbeat at this stage (some midwives won't even try to find it this early as they don't want to cause you unnecessary worry) – it should be easier to find at your next appointment, a few weeks later.

Week 13

With luck your nausea will be on the wane and you'll soon be feeling more energetic. You're probably also feeling more secure because your risk of miscarriage has now dropped dramatically. It might seem hard to believe if you're still in the throes of morning sickness, but you'll soon regain your appetite. Just make sure you're getting all the nutrients you and your baby need (see pp 52–3) and be aware of the foods that you shouldn't eat during pregnancy (see p 48).

What antenatal care will I receive?

You will have a series of antenatal check-ups throughout your pregnancy to monitor your health and your baby's development. The first, known as a booking appointment, will take place before the end of the first trimester. Your main point of contact will be a midwife, who can be contacted between antenatal checks if necessary.

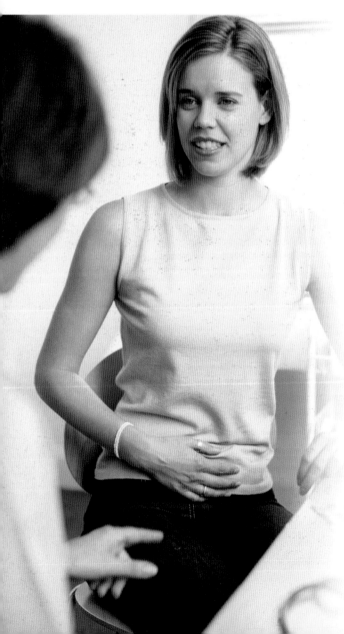

What is a booking appointment?

A booking appointment, or booking-in visit as it's also known, is your first official pregnancy check-up and takes place wherever you are going to have the bulk of your antenatal care. It provides your midwife and the rest of the team looking after you with valuable background information about your medical history and lifestyle. The term 'booking' comes from the days when women literally had to book themselves a hospital bed for labour.

When is the booking appointment?

You probably saw your doctor when you found out you were pregnant and he or she will have arranged your booking appointment. Women used to have their first antenatal appointment at 10–14 weeks, but the National Institute for Clinical Excellence (NICE) has now recommended that it takes place earlier than this. This is so that your midwife can give you information about diet and lifestyle and tell you about the various screening tests available (see pp 36–7) to give you time to decide what is best for you. This first contact may be by telephone at about 8–10 weeks, followed by a more in-depth appointment a few weeks later.

ASKING QUESTIONS *Your midwife will be able to answer any questions you have about your pregnancy. It's useful to prepare a list of any concerns before you go for the appointment.*

What happens at the first appointment?

The midwife will ask about your medical history and your lifestyle. She will take your blood pressure, measure and weigh you to work out your body mass index (see p 55), and take urine and blood samples (see pp 34–5). She may arrange for you to have a dating scan to establish the exact stage of your pregnancy. Your booking visit is a good opportunity to ask questions and discuss where you might give birth – you should be offered the chance to give birth at home if you want to.

How often will I have antenatal checks?

This will vary slightly from area to area, but the recommendation is that after the booking visit first-time mums with a straightforward pregnancy have 10 more antenatal checks at 16, 18–20, 25, 28, 31, 34, 36, 38, 40 and 41 weeks (if you haven't had your baby by then). Women who have already had a baby, and who have an uncomplicated pregnancy, should have seven checks at about 16, 18-20, 28, 34, 36, 38 and 41 weeks. If you are unhappy about long gaps between visits, talk to your midwife.

Will I always see the same midwife?

Probably not. Some areas have 'one-to-one care' under which you see the same midwife, or her back-up. Or your area may have team midwifery, where you are cared for by a group of midwives. Usually, though, you'll see a number of midwives allocated to your doctor's practice, and may not build up much of a relationship with one individual. There are no guarantees you'll have a midwife you know at the birth, but if you're being looked after by a team there's a good chance you'll have met your midwife. If you have been cared for by your practice midwife, your baby may be delivered by a hospital-based midwife who you do not know.

JUST FOR DAD

Going to antenatal appointments
Try to go to antenatal appointments as often as you can. Being by your partner's side is a great way to show your support and learn about pregnancy, birth and your developing baby. At the very least, be there for the milestones, such as the first appointment (when you'll be asked about your family health history), hearing the baby's heartbeat, the ultrasound scans and any tests.

JUST THE FACTS
QUESTIONS THE MIDWIFE WILL ASK

At the first appointment, the midwife will ask you about the following:

- **Date of last period:** *the midwife calculates your due date (see p 21) from the date of your last monthly period (LMP). You should also be offered a dating scan to get a more accurate idea of how pregnant you are and check if you are expecting more than one baby.*

- *Previous miscarriages, terminations and births: your 'obstetric history' is important and could have a bearing on how well you cope with pregnancy this time around, plus it can influence how your labour is managed.*

- *Family history of disease/genetic conditions: screening is now available for known genetic conditions such as cystic fibrosis, so if you have a family history, your midwife can explain and arrange tests. Having a family history of allergies, heart disease or certain other major medical conditions could all have a bearing on your pregnancy, so go prepared with any relevant information about both your medical history and your partner's.*

- *Your lifestyle: your midwife will ask questions such as whether you drink alcohol and smoke, and if so the quantity of each. As both can affect your baby's health, she will offer advice and put you in touch with organizations that can help with quitting. She will also ask about your diet and offer advice if needed.*

Why do I need blood and urine tests?

Your blood and urine will be tested throughout your pregnancy to monitor your health and detect potentially harmful conditions. Initial blood tests are taken to identify your blood type, check for anaemia and test for a range of infections. Urine is tested for protein and sugar content, both of which can indicate potentially serious conditions.

Why is my blood tested?

Blood tests are a routine part of your antenatal care. When you go for your booking appointment (see pp 32–3), you'll be asked to give some blood. This is to check your blood group, whether you are Rhesus positive or negative (see right), your iron levels and your immunity to rubella (German measles). Your blood is also tested for syphilis and hepatitis B.

If you have a particular reason for concern, you can also ask to be tested for toxoplasmosis and hepatitis C. All pregnant women are now offered the test for HIV/AIDS, but you don't have to have it if you don't want to. These initial blood tests are very important because they give you and your carers essential information about your health and any possible problems you might experience during your pregnancy.

What is the Rhesus factor and what happens if I'm Rhesus negative?

If you're Rhesus positive you have a certain protein on the surface of your red blood cells; if you're Rhesus negative, it isn't present. If you are Rhesus negative and your partner is positive, there's a good chance that your baby will be Rhesus positive. In this case, your body might produce antibodies that start to destroy the baby's red blood cells. If you are Rhesus negative, your blood will be tested for antibodies at 12 weeks and again at 28 weeks, and in between if you have any bleeding.

I suffer from anaemia. Will my iron levels be checked now that I'm pregnant?

Yes, a blood test can detect if your iron levels are low, which is a sign of anaemia. If you're anaemic, your doctor or midwife will talk to you about the best foods to eat (such as lean red meat and

ASK THE EXPERT
CHRISSIE HAMMONDS
MIDWIFE SONOGRAPHER

I've been told my platelet count is a little low. What does this mean?

Platelets are tiny cells that circulate round the body in the blood. They play an important role in blood clotting and fighting infection. During pregnancy it's normal for your platelet count to fall slightly, and up to eight per cent of pregnant women have platelet counts of between 100 and 150 million per millilitre of blood. This is because your body produces more of the liquid part of blood (plasma) during pregnancy, making your platelets become more dilute. This doesn't affect their performance. However, if it appears that your platelet count is lower than usual, it should be repeated so that any further reductions can be spotted. This may mean that you have a few more blood tests than other mums-to-be. The reason your platelet level is monitored is that if it becomes too low, it can affect your body's blood-clotting ability and lead to a higher risk of abnormal bleeding during or after the birth.

spinach) to boost your iron stores. You might also be prescribed iron supplements. Your iron levels will be checked again at 28 weeks, but if you suffer a lot from fatigue at any point during pregnancy, your midwife will arrange for a blood test earlier to check for anaemia.

Why is it necessary to test my blood for the hepatitis B virus?

This test is carried out because there's a small possibility you could be a carrier of the hepatitis B virus and not even know it; a blood test is often the only way to find out for certain. Your baby's liver could be seriously damaged if this disease is passed on either before or after the birth. Babies at risk of catching the hepatitis B virus from their mothers can be given injections of antibodies as soon as they are born to protect them.

What are the dangers to my baby if I'm not immune to rubella?

Most pregnant women are immune to rubella (German measles) because they've either been vaccinated against it or they've had the disease as a child. If you aren't immune, you'll be advised to avoid contact with anyone who has or might have the infection. This is because if you catch rubella during pregnancy, your baby's heart, sight and hearing could be seriously affected. You'll also be offered a vaccination after the baby is born to protect any future pregnancies.

Why is my blood tested for syphilis?

Syphilis is a sexually transmitted disease. It is fairly rare to contract it nowadays, but if you have it and it isn't treated during pregnancy, it could cause abnormalities in your developing baby. This is why it is necessary to test your blood for syphilis.

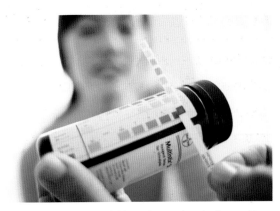

GLUCOSE TEST *A colour stick is used to test the urine for a variety of disorders. In the above case, the dark brown pad indicates a large amount of glucose in the urine, which is a positive result for diabetes.*

Why is my urine tested?

Guidelines recommend that your urine is tested early in pregnancy for bacteria because of a link between some bacteria and premature birth. Your midwife will also test your urine throughout your pregnancy for protein, which can be a sign of a urine infection or pre-eclampsia (see p 135), a potentially serious condition. You may also have your urine tested for sugar, which can be a sign of gestational diabetes.

Guidelines recommend that there is no need for every pregnant woman's urine to be tested for sugar. You may find that your urine is only tested if you fall into a high-risk group: for example, if you are overweight or you had pre-eclampsia in a previous pregnancy. If you are found to have a high level of sugar in your urine, you will also need to have a glucose tolerance test (see p 135).

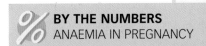

BY THE NUMBERS
ANAEMIA IN PREGNANCY

20% *The percentage of pregnant women who develop iron-deficiency anaemia in developed countries, such as the UK.*

Source: World Health Organization.

What other checks and tests will I be offered?

In addition to being given general checks to monitor your baby's well-being, in the first trimester you may be offered a dating scan at around 12 weeks and screening tests to assess the risk of Down's syndrome. The type and number of tests you're offered will depend on your age and whether your pregnancy is considered high-risk.

What is an ultrasound scan and how often will I have one?

It is now recommended that all women have a dating scan in early pregnancy to establish their baby's gestational age and detect multiple pregnancies. You may also be offered another scan at 18–20 weeks to check that your baby is developing properly, and that your placenta is positioned in a way that won't cause problems with the birth. (For more information on ultrasound, see pp 38–9.)

Will my baby's growth be monitored?

Yes. Your midwife will feel, or 'palpate', your abdomen to make sure your uterus and baby are growing properly. From around 12 weeks, she will check the baby's heartbeat with a hand-held electronic heart monitor. Once you get to about 20 weeks, she may also start measuring the size of your bump with a tape measure (from the pubic bone to the tip of your bump). This isn't a particularly accurate way of measuring, but it gives a rough idea of how your baby is progressing. Once you are near your due date, she will examine your

ASK THE EXPERT
CHRISSIE HAMMONDS
MIDWIFE SONOGRAPHER

I've been offered a nuchal translucency scan. What is it?

A nuchal translucency (NT) scan measures a collection of fluid under the skin at the back of a baby's neck. All babies have some fluid, but in many babies with Down's syndrome, the nuchal translucency is increased. The NT scan is a screening test and as such can only estimate the risk of your baby having Down's, as opposed to a diagnostic test, such as CVS (see right) or amniocentesis (see p 86), which will give you a definite diagnosis but also carries a small risk of miscarriage. NT scans are usually performed between 11 weeks and 13 weeks and six days. The results should be available immediately. If the amount of fluid is increased, it does not mean there is definitely a problem because some healthy babies can also have increased fluid.

NUCHAL TRANSLUCENCY SCAN The markers on the scan below show the area that is measured on a NT scan. A nuchal translucency measurement of up to 2 mm is normal at about 11 weeks, and up to about 2.8 mm by 13 weeks and six days.

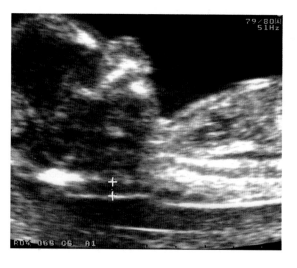

abdomen to see what position your baby is in. If she is concerned about your baby's growth and well-being, she will refer you for an ultrasound scan.

I'm 35 and having my first baby. Why is my pregnancy considered high risk?

Many recent studies have shown that in healthy women, the risks of delaying pregnancy are minimal. Actually, what's most important is the health of the mother before she conceives. That said, older women are more likely to have or develop certain medical conditions during pregnancy, such as diabetes, hypertension and placenta praevia (when the placenta lies low in the uterus, partly or completely covering the cervix). As these conditions may have serious consequences, they require closer monitoring and may place limitations on your diet and lifestyle.

Another problem is that the odds of having a baby with a genetic defect increase as you get older. For example, the risk of Down's syndrome rises from one in 885 at age 30 to one in 365 at age 35, one in 109 at age 40, and one in 32 at age 45. If you're around 40, you should strongly consider genetic testing because the risk of genetic problems increases significantly. The risk of miscarriage also increases with age. Most studies show an increased risk of Caesareans for women over 35, but the exact reasons for this are not clear.

What tests will I be offered to check for Down's Syndrome?

It's now recommended that all pregnant women are offered screening tests for Down's. In the first trimester a nuchal translucency (NT) scan (see left) can be performed at between 11 weeks and 13 weeks and six days and detects about 75 per cent of babies with Down's. There is a combined test, which is a NT scan combined with a blood test that

JUST THE FACTS
HIGH-RISK PREGNANCY

Your pregnancy may be considered high risk and require additional antenatal care if you:

- *Have previously had a pre-term delivery.*
- *Have previously had a baby with an abnormality.*
- *Are diabetic.*
- *Have high blood pressure.*
- *Are having your first baby aged over 40.*
- *Have a multiple pregnancy.*
- *Have a heart condition.*
- *Have kidney problems.*
- *Are being treated for epilepsy.*
- *Have thyroid problems.*
- *Are HIV positive.*
- *Are obese.*
- *Have an autoimmune disease, such as lupus.*
- *Are a drug/alcohol user.*
- *Have cancer.*

detects about 90 per cent of cases. This test must also be performed between 11 weeks and 13 weeks six days and is only available privately at present. There is also an integrated test, which has a 94 per cent detection rate. This involves two blood tests at about 12 and 15 weeks.

Chorionic villus sampling (CVS) is a diagnostic test that detects chromosomal abnormalities. It involves taking a tiny sample of the placenta. CVS is usually carried out between weeks 10–12. Depending on the position of the placenta or the doctor's preference, the needle is passed through the abdomen (using ultrasound for guidance), or a fine tube is threaded through the vagina and cervix to reach the placenta. There is a small risk of miscarriage with this diagnostic test (see p 87).

Ultrasound: what to expect

Seeing your baby on an ultrasound scan for the first time can be an exciting and moving experience. For many people, especially dads-to-be, it can make the pregnancy more of a reality. Scans are used to date a pregnancy and detect potential problems, but they can also provide reassurance that your baby is progressing well.

How ultrasound works

An ultrasound scan involves transmitting high frequency sound waves through the uterus. These bounce off your baby and the returning echoes are translated by a computer into an image on a screen that reveals your baby's position and movements. Hard tissues such as bone reflect the biggest echoes and are white in the image, and soft tissues appear grey and speckled. Fluids (such as the amniotic fluid that your baby lies in) do not reflect any echoes so appear black. It is the contrast between these different shades of white, grey and black that allows the images to be interpreted.

Sonographers

Ultrasound scans are usually performed by sonographers, who are radiographers or midwives specially trained in ultrasound. Special scans may be required in some pregnancies and these will be performed by a doctor trained in ultrasound, known as a Fetal Medicine Specialist.

The procedure

Having a full bladder used to be necessary for a scan, but with today's modern machines this is now rarely necessary. Ask your midwife what the policy is in your local hospital. The sonographer will put gel on your tummy and move a small hand-held transducer over your skin to get views of your baby. Sometimes a vaginal scan may be performed in early pregnancy, but this shouldn't be at all painful.

The purpose of a scan

Ultrasound scans can:
- Accurately date your pregnancy.
- Check your baby has a heartbeat.
- Check your baby's growth and development.
- Detect the number of babies.
- Detect an ectopic pregnancy (see p 18).
- Identify areas of bleeding.
- Find out why a screening test was abnormal.
- Assist in performing diagnostic tests for conditions such as Down's syndrome.
- Diagnose abnormalities, such as spina bifida.
- Assess the amount of amniotic fluid and locate the placenta.

Safety

Ultrasound was first used in pregnancy in the early 1970s, although not widely at that time. Medical research has found no side effects. No association has been shown between ultrasound exposure and the baby's birthweight, childhood leukaemias or other cancers, eyesight, hearing or dyslexia. Even so, most experts agree that the procedure shouldn't be done without clear medical reasons, and that all ultrasound exposure should be justified and limited to the minimum needed to make a diagnosis.

SEX OF THE BABY: An ultrasound scan can reveal the sex of your baby from about 18 weeks, but if your baby is lying in an awkward position it may be difficult to tell. Some hospitals have a policy of not telling women the sex of their baby, as it is not usually possible to be 100 per cent certain.

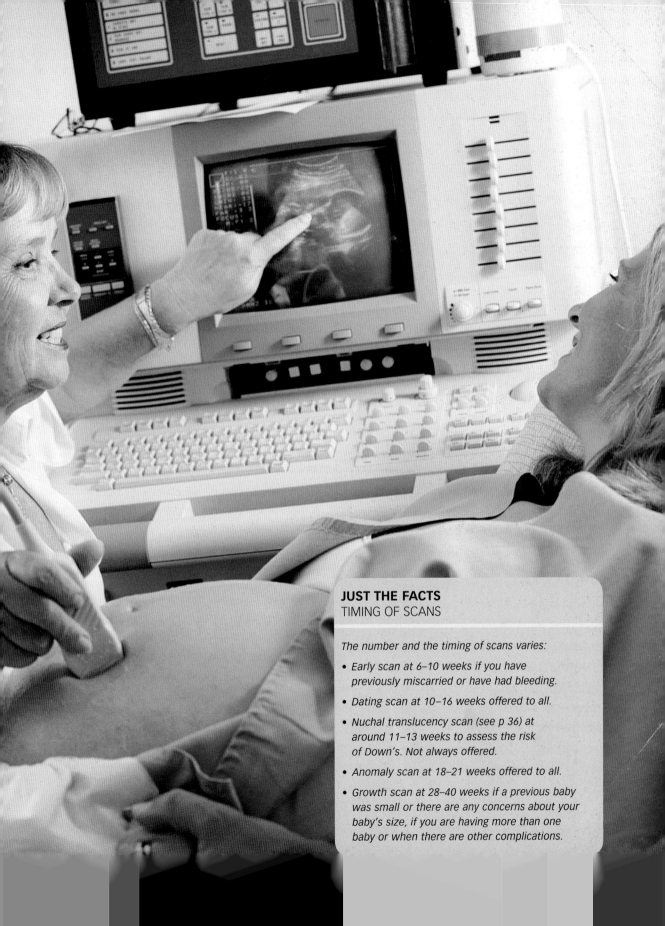

JUST THE FACTS
TIMING OF SCANS

The number and the timing of scans varies:

- *Early scan at 6–10 weeks if you have previously miscarried or have had bleeding.*

- *Dating scan at 10–16 weeks offered to all.*

- *Nuchal translucency scan (see p 36) at around 11–13 weeks to assess the risk of Down's. Not always offered.*

- *Anomaly scan at 18–21 weeks offered to all.*

- *Growth scan at 28–40 weeks if a previous baby was small or there are any concerns about your baby's size, if you are having more than one baby or when there are other complications.*

Is it normal to have sore and sensitive breasts?

Breast tenderness is one of the earliest hallmarks of pregnancy. It usually starts at around four to six weeks, lasting throughout the first trimester, and sometimes beyond. You will find that the size of your breasts gradually increases as your pregnancy progresses so you will need to invest in some new bras.

Why are my breasts so sore and sensitive to touch now that I'm pregnant?

As your body gears up for the months of pregnancy to come, it produces more of the hormones oestrogen and progesterone, just as it does before each menstrual period. In fact, the tenderness you're feeling now is probably an exaggerated version of how your breasts often feel before your period. Along with the hormone surge, your breasts are beginning to increase in size as the fat layer thickens and milk glands and extra blood are added. These changes, though temporarily uncomfortable, have an important purpose: they're preparing your breasts for feeding your baby.

Will I experience breast discomfort throughout my pregnancy?

Though your breasts will continue to grow throughout your pregnancy, they'll feel more uncomfortable in the first trimester. The size change is most noticeable in first pregnancies and any pain or discomfort associated with your breasts is likely to subside during your second and third trimesters.

The size of my breasts has increased already. How big will they grow by the end of my pregnancy?

Many women are surprised by how early they start seeing their chest grow. Breast blossoming usually begins in the first trimester, sometimes even within the first weeks of pregnancy. Most women go up at least one or two cup sizes during the course of their pregnancy; it's common to go from a B to a D cup, for example. On the other hand, don't worry if your breasts don't seem to be growing much – that's normal for some women, too, and has no bearing on your ability to breastfeed.

ASK THE EXPERT
DR MORAG MARTINDALE
GP

Why do breasts leak later in pregnancy and will it happen to me?

Possibly, but don't worry. Lots of mums-to-be find that their breasts begin to leak. Other expectant mums don't. Either way, it's normal. The liquid that leaks from your breasts is colostrum – a thick, yellowish fluid that nourishes your baby during the first few days of life. Your breasts will start to produce it around week 16 of pregnancy, but most women find they don't experience leaks until the third trimester. You may also find that your breasts leak during lovemaking, but again this is quite normal. If you do leak, it's usually only in tiny amounts. But if you find you're getting embarrassing wet patches, try wearing breast pads in your bra to protect your clothes. You can buy them in most chemists and supermarkets, and you'll need some anyway if you're planning to breastfeed. Remember to change the pads regularly during the day to keep you feeling fresh and comfortable.

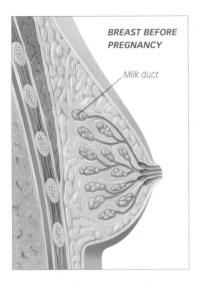

BREAST BEFORE PREGNANCY

Milk duct

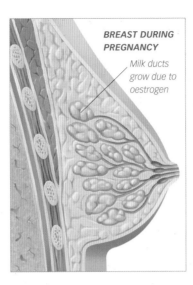

BREAST DURING PREGNANCY

Milk ducts grow due to oestrogen

BREAST CHANGES
The hormone oestrogen will lead to the growth of milk ducts in your breasts during pregnancy to prepare your body for feeding your baby. Other breast changes include dark blue veins caused by increased blood flow, the dark skin around the nipple becoming darker and the appearance of bumps around the nipples, known as Montgomery's tubercles.

My breasts are particularly sore during lovemaking. Will this pass?

It's common to experience a throb or tingle in your breasts as blood rushes to them during the initial 'excitement' phase of lovemaking. During the first trimester, you may discover that you no longer like having your breasts touched but this should pass later on in pregnancy.

What sort of bra should I wear?

It is advisable to wear a good, supportive bra. You may find that underwired bras are less comfortable now. Take the time to get fitted by a specialist, perhaps in a department store; if no one is available to help you, measure under your breasts for size and around the fullest part of your breast for the cup. If the two measurements are the same, you are an A cup. If your bust size is 2.5 cm (1 in) larger, you are a B cup, if it's 5 cm (2 in) larger you are a C cup and so on. Try to get fitted more than once during your pregnancy, as you may need to change cup sizes as your breasts grow. Cotton bras are more comfortable and breatheable than synthetic. To prevent chafing, look for soft, smooth material with

no seams near the nipple. Think carefully before buying a front-clasp bra; it may feel fine now, but as your abdomen expands, you'll find the clasp digs into your rib cage. Wear a well-fitting, supportive bra while you exercise since your breasts are heavier. Lightweight cotton sleep bras will help protect you against tenderness at night and can help prevent sagging. Buy bras that fit when the clasp is on the tightest setting, so you have room to let them out.

BabyCentre Buzz

"I wore my most comfortable bra to bed. I found that any sort of jiggling movement caused discomfort during those early weeks – so the bra stayed on 24/7." Leanne

"My breasts feel quite itchy and irritating and there's a dull ache, which makes wearing my everyday bras very uncomfortable and tight." Yvonne

"I went from a B to a C cup during my first pregnancy, then went back to normal after weaning. My breasts stayed small when I was pregnant with my second. They may not have grown much, but they certainly made plenty of milk!" Marie

I feel really tired. Will it last?

Growing a new human being is very tiring work, making fatigue one of the most common symptoms of early pregnancy. Unfortunately, there is no cure for it. You simply have to wait for it to pass (it usually does by the second trimester), and in the meantime adapt your lifestyle so that you get the maximum amount of rest.

Why am I so tired now that I'm pregnant?

What many women remember most about the early stages of pregnancy is that constant feeling of fatigue. Even night owls find themselves struggling to stay awake. Throughout pregnancy, but especially in the first trimester, your body works tremendously hard. Your body is making the placenta, and your hormone levels and metabolism are changing while your blood sugar and blood pressure may be lower. All these factors contribute to a sense of fatigue.

Am I going to feel this tired throughout my pregnancy?

It's different for everyone, but pregnant women usually experience fatigue in the first trimester and at the beginning of the second trimester, but then begin to gradually regain their energy. Once your baby is born, you may well look back on this period of undisturbed nights with nostalgia. So consider stocking up on your sleep if you can (it may not be that easy if you already have children or if you work full-time). It's common to begin to run out of steam again around the seventh month of pregnancy.

I start feeling drowsy at about 8 o'clock in the evening. Is this normal?

Yes, this is a very common symptom of early pregnancy and you shouldn't fight it. Your body is sending you a message that you (and your baby) need more sleep. It's better to turn in earlier than you're accustomed to than to doze off on the couch. That way, you're likely to get a longer stretch of uninterrupted sleep – instead of waking up hours later and having to turn out the lights and drag yourself to bed, where you may find yourself staring at the ceiling, willing yourself back to sleep.

I'm worn out during the day but then don't seem to be able to sleep that well once I go to bed. What can I do?

It depends what's keeping you awake. If you're having to get up to go to the toilet, limit what you drink before bedtime and cut down on caffeinated drinks during the day – they are diuretics and will make you want to urinate more frequently. When you do go to the toilet, lean forward slightly to ensure you have completely emptied your bladder. If digestive problems (see pp 144–5) are the problem, avoid eating fatty foods at dinnertime as these take

QUICK TIP

Don't rely on quick pick-me-ups such as caffeine and chocolate – they may give you a temporary energy boost, but you'll crash quickly and hard. Snacking on healthy foods such as fruit and yoghurt will give you energy without making you feel sluggish.

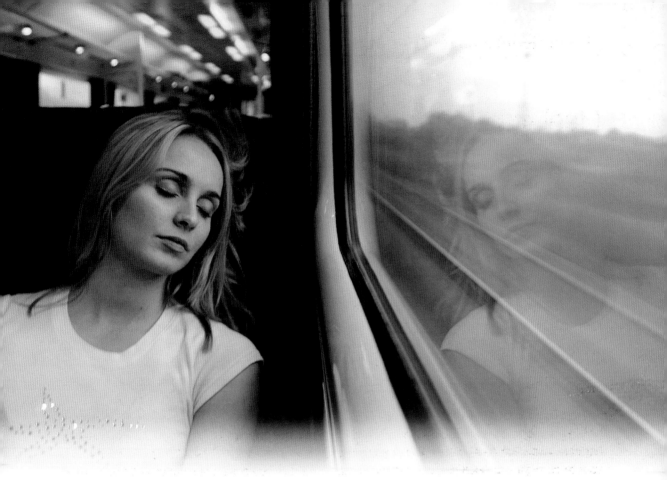

CATNAPS To cope with pregnancy fatigue, you'll need to make the most of every opportunity you can to snooze. If you have to commute to work, the tiredness can be even worse so make sure you ask for a seat on a public transport.

longer to digest and steer clear of rich, spicy, acidic or fried foods. If you're feeling nauseous during the night, keep some simple snacks, such as crackers, on your bedside table. Some women find it difficult to get comfortable because of breast tenderness (see pp 40–41). If this is the problem, try wearing a soft cotton bra at night and train yourself to sleep on your side. You'll need to do this later in pregnancy anyway (see p 94).

I'm often really sleepy during the day. Should I take catnaps?

It's very common in early pregnancy to start feeling sleepy during the day. This sudden craving for naps may be caused by increasing levels of progesterone, a pregnancy hormone that has a sedative effect.

Unfortunately, there's no way around this problem other than to rest as much as you can and grab a quick catnap whenever possible. Keep in mind, though, that napping too late in the day (or for more than 30 to 60 minutes) can disrupt a good night's sleep. If you work, you may have to resort to going to a staffroom or even sleeping in your car in your lunch hour. If napping isn't an option, going for a gentle walk may help to revive you.

IF YOU DO NOTHING ELSE...

- *Listen to your body's signals and take catnaps whenever you can.*
- *Try to adjust your schedule so that you get some rest.*
- *Learn to say 'no' to people and put yourself first.*
- *Make sure you're eating properly (see pp 48–9).*
- *Forget the housework.*

What causes morning sickness and what can I do to relieve it?

Nausea or vomiting during pregnancy is thought to be caused by hormonal changes. Most women quickly learn what is most likely to trigger the sickness and find simple ways to manage it until it passes, usually at the beginning of the second trimester.

If it's called morning sickness, why do I feel sick all day long?

Like most pregnant women, you've discovered that so-called 'morning sickness' can strike morning, noon or night. There's no single explanation for why you're feeling sick. Some combination of the many physical changes taking place in your body is probably responsible. Those changes include rapidly increasing oestrogen levels, an enhanced sense of smell, excess stomach acids and increased fatigue. Some researchers theorize that stress and emotions may also play a role in morning sickness. Although it won't alleviate your nausea, it may be reassuring to

know you're not alone. About 75–80 per cent of mums-to-be find the early weeks of pregnancy feel like one long, sickening ride on a rollercoaster. It can also be difficult to cope with morning sickness at work (see pp 68–9).

Am I likely to feel nauseous throughout my pregnancy?

No two pregnancies are alike, and the same goes for bouts of morning sickness. The nausea you're feeling can last anywhere from a few weeks to a few months – or longer, though that's rare. By the end of the third month, most women stop feeling nauseous. Unfortunately, queasiness or mild nausea can come and go throughout pregnancy. It's often brought on by certain smells, but the triggers vary from woman to woman.

Will morning sickness affect my baby?

Morning sickness won't threaten your developing baby's wellbeing as long as you're able to keep food down, eat a well-balanced diet and drink plenty of fluids. Most women with morning sickness work out pretty quickly what they can and cannot stomach, and how many times they need to eat throughout the day. Experiment to find out what works for you. If your morning sickness is so severe that you really can't keep anything down (see right), seek medical advice.

BabyCentre Buzz

"Peppermint oil really helps my sickness. When I feel nauseated, I just hold it to my nose and sniff." Valerie

"When I don't get enough sleep, I feel horrible the whole next day. When I do sleep, my morning sickness is more manageable." Karen

"Lemon ice-lollies really eased my nausea. Friends who've been truly ill have even tried sucking on a lemon itself." Wendy

"I've found that sucking on a peppermint sweet helps. I carry them round with me all the time." Amanda

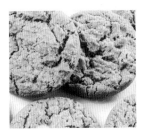
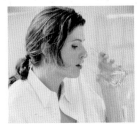

STOMACH SETTLERS *Nibbling a ginger biscuit may settle your stomach. Stick to plain drinks – a glass of water is often best.*

Do antenatal supplements help or hinder morning sickness?

Taking antenatal supplements (see p 49) can sometimes make nausea in pregnancy worse, so try discontinuing them temporarily. If the nausea improves, give yourself a few days off and then try taking them again. Since iron can be hard on your digestive system, don't take iron supplements unless a blood test shows that you are anaemic (see p 34). Even then, it's worth trying different brands as some may suit you better than others. If you find antenatal vitamins hard to keep down, try taking them with food. If you still can't stomach them, consider eating a vitamin-fortified cereal every morning. And make sure you eat a diet that's rich in all the vitamins you and your developing baby need (see pp 52–3).

I'm vomiting so often I just can't keep anything down. What should I do?

Talk to your doctor immediately as you may have the rare condition hyperemesis gravidarum (literally 'excessive vomiting in pregnancy'). As frightening as it sounds, it can be treated. If left untreated, excessive vomiting can lead to malnutrition, dehydration and other complications for you and your baby. Your doctor or midwife can help you by prescribing a special diet, suggesting you rest in bed, or even admitting you to hospital. If you're

diagnosed as dehydrated, you may be hospitalized to be given fluids via a drip. You may also be given medication to decrease your nausea and vomiting and help you to keep food down.

What is an acupressure band and how does it help morning sickness?

This is a simple device, created to help prevent seasickness, that has helped many pregnant women through morning sickness. Strap it on so that the plastic button pushes against an acupressure point in your wrist, and you may begin to feel some relief from your nausea. Acupressure bands are available from chemists.

JUST THE FACTS
TRIED AND TESTED REMEDIES

To prevent – or at least minimize – queasiness you may want to try the following:

- *Keep plain biscuits or crackers by your bed. Nibble a few and then rest before getting out of bed.*

- *Eat small, frequent meals as an empty stomach can increase nausea. Foods high in protein or complex carbohydrates help to fight nausea.*

- *Try to avoid rich, spicy, acidic or fried foods, and eat less fat in general.*

- *It's important to stay hydrated, but try drinking fluids only between meals, and limit them during meals.*

- *Even though you may not be able to stomach big meals, snacking on bland food throughout the day may make you feel better. Good choices include dry biscuits and yoghurt.*

- *Sniff lemons. The smell of a cut lemon may help your nausea. Add some slices to iced tea or sparkling water.*

- *Drink ginger tea or eat ginger biscuits. Ginger is known to settle stomachs and help queasiness.*

How will my pregnancy differ if I'm expecting more than one baby?

Because you're expecting more than one baby, your pregnancy is considered higher-risk and will be monitored more closely. Don't, however, assume you'll develop complications. Most multiple pregnancies are straightforward.

How will my antenatal care differ?

Your doctors and midwives will monitor you carefully, and they will work with you to ensure that your pregnancy goes as close to full-term as possible. Roughly half of all twins are delivered before week 37, but unless and until there is an overwhelming reason to deliver early, keep your goal of going the distance firmly in mind. Expect to have more antenatal appointments – usually every 2–3 weeks in the first and second trimesters, and then weekly in the third trimester. Besides monitoring your health, your obstetrician will want to keep a close eye on your babies' growth. As it is difficult to determine how well your babies are growing by feeling your tummy, you will be offered extra scans. If your twins are identical and therefore share a placenta, you'll have more frequent checks and scans, including one to check for twin-to-twin transfusion, which occurs when one twin gets more than its fair share of the circulating blood.

If you are carrying triplets, which are less common than twins, your antenatal care and delivery should be in a big consultant-led unit.

Will I have more complications?

You won't necessarily have any pregnancy complications if you are expecting twins. However, unfortunately, the rate of miscarriage (see pp 18–19) is higher if you are carrying more than one baby, and particularly if your babies are identical (when one fertilized egg divides in half). As with a single pregnancy, most miscarriages in multiple pregnancies happen in the first 12 weeks. Sometimes only one baby is lost. In this case, the risk of anything happening to your remaining baby is low. Getting an early confirmation that you are carrying more than one baby will give your carers plenty of time to detect and treat any complications. Triplets are less common than twins

ASK THE EXPERT
DR MAGGIE BLOTT
CONSULTANT OBSTETRICIAN

Can I still have a nuchal translucency scan if I'm expecting twins?

Yes, a nuchal translucency (NT) scan (see p 36) is the best screening test for Down's syndrome when you are having twins. The blood screening test that is normally offered in a single pregnancy does not work as well for a multiple pregnancy. A NT scan will measure the fluid at the back of both babies' necks so that each can be given its individual risk. Before deciding whether or not to have a NT scan for twins, you need to think about what you would do if one baby has a high risk and one a low. The only way to know for sure if your babies are healthy is to have a diagnostic test, such as amniocentesis (see p 86), and the risk of miscarriage following these is doubled with twins. If only one baby is affected, you may be faced with a difficult decision. If the twins are identical they will either both have Down's or neither will have it.

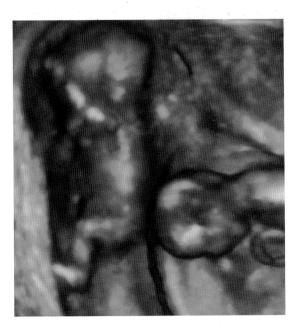

POSITION IN THE UTERUS *It is common for one baby to lie in a breech position in a twin pregnancy. If the breech baby doesn't turn, it may reduce the chances of delivering your babies naturally. This 3-D scan picture shows twins in early pregnancy.*

but are associated with increased complications. Triplets are much more likely to be delivered prematurely, often as early as 26-28 weeks.

Will my pregnancy symptoms be worse?

Yes, unfortunately. The usual symptoms are likely to be more severe, particularly morning sickness (see pp 44–5). Other common problems include an inability to sleep, fatigue (see pp 42–3), general discomfort and achiness, swollen hands and feet (see pp 92–3). You are also likely to find it slightly more difficult to move around in later pregnancy.

Do I need to adapt my diet even more for a multiple pregnancy?

There are no specific guidelines on nutrition for a multiple pregnancy. As in a single pregnancy, the recommendation is that you eat to satisfy your appetite and ensure that you have a healthy, varied diet (see pp 48–9). Eating well will increase the odds that you'll have babies that are a healthy weight. As your pregnancy advances, you may find that you can't easily digest large meals and prefer to eat little and often. Anaemia (see pp 34–5) is more common in women carrying more than one child, so your midwife will check your blood regularly and advise you to take iron supplements if necessary.

Can I deliver my twins naturally?

There is some evidence that it may be safer to deliver twins by Caesarean, especially for the second twin. Also, it's much more common for one of the babies to be lying in the breech position in a multiple pregnancy. For these reasons the majority of twins, but not all, are delivered by Caesarean. However, many women are able to have vaginal births. Talk to your doctor about the policy in your local hospital and the options available to you.

You're more likely to be able to deliver your babies naturally if your pregnancy has been normal, and if your babies are growing well and lying in a good position. If you do opt to have a normal delivery, many maternity units will suggest that you have an epidural (see pp 174–5) during labour and that your babies are continually monitored.

Your chances of needing an emergency Caesarean during labour is higher with a multiple pregnancy, and there is also an increased chance that you'll need to have a forceps or ventouse delivery (see pp 190–91).

 QUICK TIP

Drinking plenty of fluids is even more crucial when you're carrying more than one baby; the risk of having premature contractions, and an early delivery, increases if you become dehydrated. Aim to drink a minimum of eight glasses of water a day.

What should I be eating now that I'm pregnant?

It can be difficult to eat a balanced diet during pregnancy if you're battling waves of nausea brought on by morning sickness. But to stay healthy and fuel your baby's development, it is important to try and eat a healthy, varied diet that contains a wide range of vitamins and minerals.

My diet is already quite good. Do I need to change it now that I'm pregnant?

Even if you already eat well, it's important to fine-tune your diet now that you're a mum-to-be. Try to increase your intake of certain vitamins and minerals, such as folic acid (found in dark green leafy vegetables), iron (found in pulses, green vegetables and fortified breakfast cereals) and

JUST THE FACTS
FOODS TO AVOID DURING PREGNANCY

During pregnancy you should avoid eating:

- *Raw seafood, such as oysters or uncooked sushi.*

- *Shark, swordfish and marlin.*

- *Cheeses with a white, 'mouldy' rind, such as Brie and Camembert, and blue-veined cheeses.*

- *Pâté, raw or undercooked meat, poultry and eggs (cook all meat until there are no pink bits, and eggs until they are hard). All are possible sources of bacteria that can harm your baby.*

- *Liver and liver products (pâté, liver sausage) because they may contain large amounts of the retinol form of vitamin A, too much of which could be bad for your developing baby.*

- *Avoid peanuts and foods that contain them if you, your partner, or any of your other children have a history of allergies. This can help to prevent your baby developing a peanut allergy.*

calcium (found in dairy foods and sesame seeds). Aside from that, just double-check that your diet is varied enough to provide all the key nutrients that will benefit your unborn baby's health (see pp 52–3).

I've lost my appetite since becoming pregnant. Is this normal and will it last?

In the first few weeks your appetite may fall away dramatically and you may not feel like eating proper meals, especially if you suffer from nausea or sickness. During the middle part of your pregnancy your appetite may be the same as before you were pregnant or slightly increased. Towards the end of your pregnancy your appetite will probably increase, but you may want to eat little and often because of heartburn and indigestion (see p 144). The best rule to remember is eat when you are hungry. Don't worry about your changing appetite as long as you are following the advice given about the type of food you need to eat and your baby is growing well.

Can I still eat fast food and have an occasional sweet treat?

You don't have to give up all your favourite foods but do try to limit junk food, as it offers little more than empty calories (calories with few or no nutrients) and make sure processed foods, snacks and sugar-packed desserts aren't the mainstay of your diet. As far as snacks are concerned, try

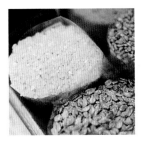 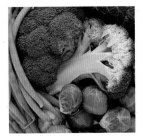 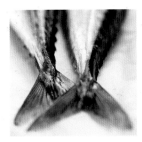 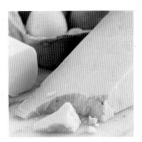

GET THE BALANCE RIGHT *To get the nutrients you need during pregnancy, include all the main food groups in your diet – grains, fruit and vegetables, well-cooked meat, fish and poultry, and dairy products.*

a banana rather than ice cream, or a frozen fruit sorbet instead of canned peaches in sugary syrup. But don't feel guilty if you fancy the occasional biscuit. Enjoy every bite!

Should I be taking an antenatal supplement?

In an ideal world – free of morning sickness or food aversions – a well-balanced diet would be all an expectant mum ever needed. But in the real world, a vitamin-mineral supplement may be good insurance that a pregnant woman will be able to meet her nutritional needs. Remember, however, that it can be just as harmful having too many supplements as too few. Seek advice from your doctor or pharmacist about which vitamin supplement to take.

I'm taking a supplement but I keep being sick. What should I do?

Take your supplement with a meal or snack to reduce the chances of being sick. If you feel particularly nauseous in the morning, take your supplement later in the day or at bedtime, or try breaking it in half and taking each part a few hours apart. If all else fails, stop taking it for a while and make sure your diet is providing the basic nutrients you need (see above). Mention the sickness to your midwife at your next antenatal appointment.

I can't stomach fruit and vegetables. What can I do?

Try drinking your fruit and vegetables in the form of juice. You could buy a juicer or blender and make your own. If all else fails, take an antenatal supplement and try fruit and veg again in a few weeks when your stomach may have settled.

Do I need to adapt my vegetarian diet?

Your body requires a little more protein during pregnancy, and this is easily provided by following a healthy, varied vegetarian diet. However, you should ensure you have an adequate intake of iron and calcium. Try to have some food or drink containing vitamin C with any iron-rich meals to help absorption. Avoid consuming caffeine with iron-rich foods as this reduces absorption. The best sources of calcium are dairy foods. Aim to have three servings per day. If you do not eat dairy foods, then it is a good idea to take a supplement.

IF YOU DO NOTHING ELSE...

- *Eat a balanced diet.*
- *Stay hydrated.*
- *Eat small amounts rather than nothing at all.*
- *Seek medical advice if you can't keep food down.*

Can I drink whatever I want?

Staying hydrated during pregnancy helps to ease pregnancy niggles, such as piles, constipation and fluid retention. Try to always keep a bottle of water to hand and limit caffeinated and high-sugar drinks. If you choose not to stop drinking alcohol, make sure you follow the recommended guidelines for alcohol intake.

Is it safe to drink herbal teas?

You can drink herbal teas but do be cautious. While many women avoid all drugs during pregnancy, including caffeine, alcohol, nicotine and medicines, they often think nothing of drinking cup after cup of herbal tea. Remember that herbs are drugs – often powerful ones. In some cultures women actually take herbal potions to terminate pregnancies. High doses of some herbs may cause diarrhoea, vomiting and heart palpitations, especially if you drink too much.

Although no food regulations in the UK specifically address herbal teas, any herb considered fine for food use is presumed to be safe for teas as well. All herbal preparations bought in the form of a tea bag are considered safe for pregnancy. In the USA, women are advised to limit their consumption to two 226 g (8 oz) servings per day. If you enjoy herbal teas, look on the label for contents that may normally be part of your diet (such as mint or orange extracts) and steer clear of unfamiliar ingredients (such as cohosh, pennyroyal and mugwort, all best avoided during pregnancy).

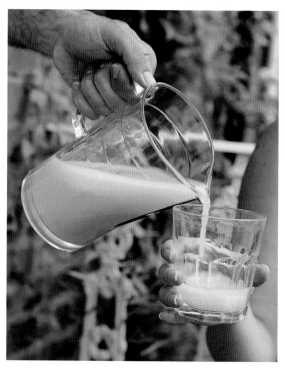

REFRESHING AND HEALTHY Fruit juices make a refreshing change to drinking water, and have the added advantage of providing you with an intake of healthy vitamins.

You could consider making your own concoction using juices, lemon rinds, cinnamon, ginger, or other ingredients, along with boiled water or decaffeinated tea. Never make a tea from any plant in your own garden, unless you're 100 per cent sure what it is and that you can safely take it while you're pregnant.

QUICK TIP

If you don't like the taste of plain water, try adding a wedge of lemon or lime or a splash of juice for flavour. Sparkling water – flavoured or unflavoured – is also a good alternative.

I'm a caffeine addict. Can I still start the day with a cup of coffee?

Yes, you can still enjoy your favourite caffeinated drinks as long as you don't overdo it. Guidelines issued by the Food Standards Agency suggest that women have no more than 300 mg of caffeine a day while pregnant. This is equivalent to three mugs of instant coffee, six cups of tea or eight cans of cola per day. Moderate amounts of caffeine are unlikely to harm you or your unborn baby, but some women choose to cut out caffeine completely, switch to non-caffeinated drinks or cut down by switching from fresh to instant coffee and brewing their tea for slightly less time. Don't forget chocolate also contains caffeine and some high-energy drinks contain quite large amounts too.

Is it safe to use artificial sweeteners?

Aspartame, an artificial sweetener found in many diet soft drinks, is considered safe in pregnancy, although the Food Standards Agency (see p 227) recommends that adults do not exceed a daily intake of 2,800 mg. This is equivalent to about 14 cans of a diet drink per day! Saccharin, another artificial sweetener found commonly in foods and drinks, is also considered safe for pregnant women. The main health issue for pregnant women who use artificial sweeteners is that they may be missing out on more nutritious foods and drinks. A woman who drinks a lot of diet cola, for instance, may not be getting enough water, milk or juice, which are all beneficial to her developing baby, or she may be consuming too much caffeine.

Is it okay to have alcohol occasionally?

The truth is we don't really know what a safe level of alcohol consumption is for a pregnant woman – and it's probably different for every woman

BabyCentre Buzz

"When everyone around you is drinking champagne to make a special toast to someone, drink sparkling apple or grapefruit juice – but put it in the champagne glass. You won't feel left out then." Denise

"I'm a Virgin Mary fan – it's a Bloody Mary with the tomato juice, a dash of Worcestershire sauce, a dash of Tabasco and a twist of lemon, but no vodka. It's really delicious." Martine

"Mix some orange juice, a good-sized splash of cranberry juice, a small splash of grapefruit juice or pineapple juice – and a dash of grenadine for sweetness if you like." Elaine

because everyone metabolizes alcohol differently. The effects of alcohol are greater on women who smoke, consume large amounts of caffeine and have a poor diet. Some health experts recommend that pregnant women play it safe by steering clear of alcohol altogether. The Royal College of Obstetricians and Gynaecologists recommends that women should be careful about alcohol consumption in pregnancy and limit their intake to no more than one unit of alcohol per day (equal to one small glass of wine). The Food Standards Agency (see p 227) advises having no more than one or two alcoholic drinks once or twice per week.

I didn't realize I was pregnant and got drunk. Could I have harmed my baby?

This is a common concern because most women don't realize they're pregnant in the first few weeks. It's unlikely that having one alcoholic drink too many on a single occasion will have affected your unborn baby, but keep track of how much alcohol you're drinking from now on, following the guidelines that are outlined above.

Nutrients you need to help your baby grow

NUTRIENT	RDA (RECOMMENDED DAILY AMOUNT)	FUNCTION	GOOD SOURCES
CALCIUM	800 mg	Helps your baby develop strong bones and teeth, healthy nerves, heart and muscles. Also develops heart rhythm and blood clotting.	• Dairy foods eg. milk and yoghurt • Spinach and other green vegetables • Beans and sesame seeds • Dried fruit • White flour products • Fortified breakfast cereals
COPPER	1.2 mg	Helps form a baby's heart, skeletal and nervous systems, and blood vessels.	• Green vegetables • Fish, liver and nuts • Cereals and cereal products.
IRON	14.8 mg	Benefits your baby by making red blood cells, supplying oxygen to cells for energy and growth, and building bones and teeth.	• Meat, especially red meat • Pilchards • Beans and lentils • Eggs • Nuts • Bread, fortified breakfast cereals, pasta and chapatti • Green vegetables and dried fruit
MAGNESIUM	70 mg	Helps your baby develop strong bones and teeth, regulates insulin and blood-sugar levels; builds and repairs tissue.	• Green leafy vegetables (such as spinach) and nuts • Bread • Fish and meat • Dairy foods eg. milk and yoghurt
ZINC	7 mg	Important for growth, wound healing and in the body's immune system.	• Lean meats and poultry • Eggs and dairy products • Whole grains • Beans and nuts
FOLIC ACID	300 mcg plus 400 mcg supplement before conception and for the first three months of pregnancy	Helps reduce the risk of neural tube defects such as spina bifida. Also helps to form red blood cells.	• Green leafy vegetables • Peas and chickpeas • Yeast extract • Brown rice • Oranges and bananas • Fortified cereals and bread

NUTRIENT	RDA (RECOMMENDED DAILY AMOUNT)	FUNCTION	GOOD SOURCES
RIBOFLAVIN	1.14 mg	Promotes growth, good vision, and healthy skin. Essential for your baby's bone, muscle, and nerve development.	• Dairy products and eggs • Meats and kidneys • Mushrooms and green vegetables, • Yeast and meat extract • Enriched bread and cereals
THIAMIN	0.9 mg	Converts carbs into energy; essential for your baby's brain development.	• Pork • Meat and yeast extract (Marmite) • Eggs and milk • White bread and breakfast cereals
VITAMIN A	700 mcg	Important for cell growth, eye development and infection resistance.	• Offal (pregnant women should not eat liver or liver products) • Egg yolk • Butter and margarine • Carrots • Green vegetables
VITAMIN B6	0.96 mg	Aids metabolism of protein, fats and carbs. Helps form red blood cells and develop brain and nervous system.	• Bananas and watermelon • Broccoli and spinach • Red meat • Fish • Poultry
VITAMIN C	50 mg	Essential for tissue repair and collagen production. Helps growth and strengthens bones and teeth.	• Most fruits and vegetables • Some of the richest are green peppers, cauliflower, broccoli, cabbage, strawberries, citrus fruits and potatoes.
VITAMIN D	10 mcg	Helps build bones and teeth.	• In the UK, being outside in the sunshine for short periods between 11 am and 3 pm during the summer should provide enough stores of Vitamin D to last through the winter months. • Dietary sources are oily fish, eggs, fortified margarine and milk.
VITAMIN B12	1.5 mcg	For red blood cells and nerve cell formation.	• Red meats • Milk • Eggs

How much weight will I gain during pregnancy?

Many women worry about piling on the weight during pregnancy, but it's important to accept that you're going to do so. You're meant to because your body is changing to give your baby the best start in life. Be reassured that your midwife will keep an eye on your weight gain. Talk to her if you have concerns.

Will I be weighed at all of my antenatal appointments?

No. Not so long ago, pregnant women used to be weighed at every antenatal check. Then doctors realized that this made a lot of women very anxious and, in any case, wasn't a particularly good way of assessing how well the pregnancy was progressing. They also realized that weight gain in pregnancy

should be related to a woman's Body Mass Index (BMI) before she became pregnant. For this reason, it's now recommended that your midwife calculates your BMI (see right) at your booking appointment (see p 32) and monitors your weight gain in relation to this.

Should I be aiming to eat a certain number of calories per day?

You don't need to be eating extra calories until later on in your pregnancy (see pp 102–3). What's more important than counting calories is eating a sensible diet that includes foods from all the major food groups. About 10 per cent of your calories should come from proteins, such as meat, fish, eggs and pulses. About 35 per cent of your calories should come from dairy products, such as butter and cheese, and from oils and nuts (fats). About 55 per cent of your calories (the largest part) should come from bread, pasta, potatoes, rice and cereals (carbohydrates).

I've always been overweight and am constantly trying to lose it. Is it okay to diet while I'm pregnant?

It's not a good idea to go on a diet during pregnancy. If you're already overweight you should try to limit the amount of weight you gain because piling on the weight could increase your risk of

ASK THE EXPERT
FIONA FORD
DIETICIAN

I've been battling an eating disorder for about 10 years. Will it affect my unborn baby?

It is particularly important to get help with your pregnancy weight and nutrition goals if you have an eating disorder. Not only are you and your unborn baby at greater risk of pregnancy complications, but you may also need assistance to break unhealthy eating patterns that may have been a part of your life for years. If you're underweight when you conceive your baby, you may be starting out with a nutritional disadvantage, since you're likely to have inadequate stores of fat for pregnancy.

Some studies have linked being underweight at conception to an increased risk of premature birth and low birthweight. However, other studies show that there is no risk if you gain enough weight during your pregnancy. So work closely with your carers to map out a healthy weight-gain and eating plan. You may be referred to a nutritionist for specialist help.

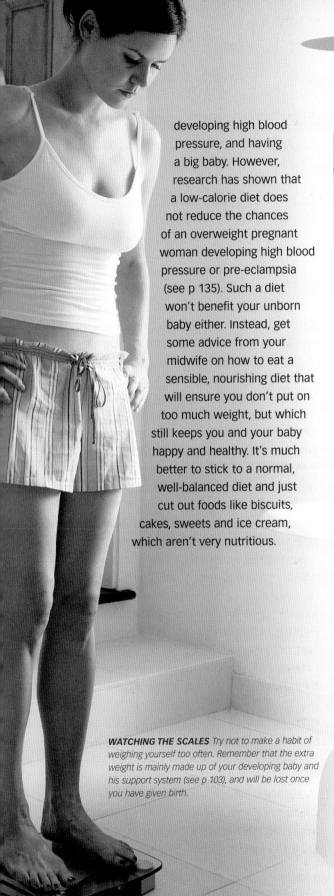

developing high blood pressure, and having a big baby. However, research has shown that a low-calorie diet does not reduce the chances of an overweight pregnant woman developing high blood pressure or pre-eclampsia (see p 135). Such a diet won't benefit your unborn baby either. Instead, get some advice from your midwife on how to eat a sensible, nourishing diet that will ensure you don't put on too much weight, but which still keeps you and your baby happy and healthy. It's much better to stick to a normal, well-balanced diet and just cut out foods like biscuits, cakes, sweets and ice cream, which aren't very nutritious.

WATCHING THE SCALES Try not to make a habit of weighing yourself too often. Remember that the extra weight is mainly made up of your developing baby and his support system (see p 103), and will be lost once you have given birth.

JUST THE FACTS
CALCULATING YOUR BODY MASS INDEX (BMI)

1. Multiply your height in metres by your height in metres. If you are 1.6 m (5 ft 3 in) multiply 1.6 by 1.6 which gives you 2.56.

2. Then divide your weight in kg by this figure. So, if you weigh 60 kg (132 lb), your BMI will be 60 divided by 2.56 = 23.43.

BMI less than 20	– Underweight
BMI 20–25	– Ideal
BMI 25–30	– Overweight
BMI 30–40	– Obese
BMI greater than 40	– Severely obese

Your BMI and pregnancy weight gain
In the 1990s, the Institute of Medicine in the USA recommended that women should aim for a weight gain related to their pre-pregnancy BMI:

- Aim for a weight gain of 6.35 kg (14 lb) if you were overweight before you became pregnant.

- Aim for a weight gain of 12.7 kg (28 lb) if you were a normal weight before you became pregnant.

- Aim for a weight gain of 19 kg (42 lb) if you were underweight before you became pregnant.

Note: If you're under 20 years of age, you should aim for a weight gain at the top end of the range for someone with your pre-pregnancy BMI.

If I gain a lot of weight during my pregnancy, does it mean I'll have a bigger baby?

No. The size of your newborn baby will be determined mainly by the size of you and your partner. It can also be influenced by medical conditions during pregnancy, such as diabetes (see p 135), and by lifestyle factors such as smoking (see pp 14–15).

Should I be exercising during pregnancy?

Moderate exercise will get you in good shape for labour and can help to ease some pregnancy discomforts. But remember that your body has changed: your centre of gravity has shifted, you're carrying more weight and you'll tire more quickly. That's why it's important to exercise with care and listen to your body.

Which forms of exercise are best for pregnant women?

Ideal exercise gets your heart pumping, keeps you supple, manages weight gain and prepares your muscles for the hard work of labour and delivery – without causing undue physical stress to you or your baby. Walking, jogging, swimming, stationary cycling and aquanatal workouts are all considered good, safe exercises during pregnancy, as long as you ensure you don't overdo it. Yoga and Pilates (see pp 146–7) are good, as long as you find a registered practitioner who is experienced in dealing with pregnant women.

Which activities are not recommended?

Avoid contact sports with a high potential for hard falls or ones where you might be thrown off-balance. These include horse-riding, downhill skiing, gymnastics and waterskiing. Scuba-diving is unsafe at any stage of pregnancy. Additionally, it is recommended that you give up cycling after the second trimester, even if you're experienced, because of the potential for falls. You can, however, use an exercise bike for as long as you want.

What are the benefits of exercising during pregnancy?

Exercise does wonders for you during pregnancy. It helps prepare you for childbirth by strengthening your muscles and building endurance, and makes getting your body back in shape once your baby is born much easier. It can also help with back pain and some research suggests that it may help to make your labour shorter. Staying active during pregnancy doesn't necessarily mean going for the burn. Your body releases a hormone called relaxin during pregnancy that loosens your joints in preparation for delivery, so you need to take

JUST THE FACTS
RISK FACTORS

Seek medical advice before exercising if you:

- *Have had a threatened miscarriage.*
- *Have had a previous premature baby or are at risk of premature labour.*
- *Know that you have a low-lying placenta.*
- *Have had significant bleeding.*
- *Have had lower back or hip problems.*
- *Have a pre-existing medical condition.*
- *Have very high blood pressure.*
- *Are expecting more than one baby.*
- *Are anaemic (have low iron in your blood).*
- *Are expecting a small-for-dates baby.*
- *Are very underweight or have an eating disorder.*
- *Have a weak or incompetent cervix.*

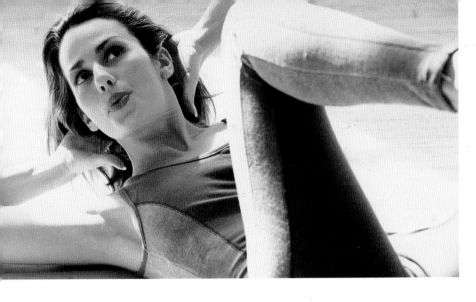

EXERCISE CLASSES You can continue to go to exercise classes, but tell the instructor that you are expecting a baby. Ideally, find a class that is aimed at pregnant women. For variety, look out for pregnancy aquanatal classes.

care with your choice of exercise and pay attention to technique. It's important to find exercises that won't injure you or harm your baby. Being active during your pregnancy can also reduce the physical discomforts of backache, constipation, fatigue and swelling, as well as improve your mood and self-image; it can even help you sleep more soundly.

I haven't exercised for years. Are there any special precautions I should take?

Pregnancy is not the time to take up a new high-impact and strenuous sport, but as long as you get the go-ahead from your midwife or doctor, you can engage in mild to moderate exercise. Stick to low-impact activities such as walking or swimming, and keep workouts short. Make sure that you warm up before exercising and cool down afterwards. It is also advisable to join a specific pregnancy or antenatal exercise class.

What's the danger of getting overheated?

Although there's no proof of a danger to humans, some animal studies suggest that overheating, especially in the early months of pregnancy, can cause birth defects. To be on the safe side, avoid overheating through exercise, especially in the first trimester. Sauna and jacuzzi use in early pregnancy – which also raises body temperature – has been shown to increase birth defects, so avoid them

completely. Your temperature (taken under the arm) should be less than 38.3°C (101°F) after exercising. To stay cool, don't exercise for long periods if it's hot or humid outside, wear proper workout clothes and drink plenty of fluids. Dehydration raises body temperature so drink about half a litre (a pint) of water or a sports drink two hours before you begin exercising. During your workout, drink another glass or two of water every 15 to 20 minutes.

Can I continue my high-intensity workouts now that I'm pregnant?

If you're in good health, quite fit, and feel up to it, go ahead and continue. According to a recent study in the *American Journal of Obstetrics and Gynecology*, healthy, well-conditioned women who exercised before pregnancy can continue to do so without compromising their baby's health.

IF YOU DO NOTHING ELSE...

- *Seek medical advice if you are new to exercise.*
- *Follow the guidelines for which exercises are recommended during pregnancy.*
- *Drink water before, during and after exercise.*
- *Listen to your body and stop exercising if you begin to feel unwell.*

I'm really happy so why do I keep having mood swings?

You will probably experience a range of emotions in the early weeks, from excitement and anticipation to anxiety and irritability. It's normal for feelings to fluctuate at this stage of pregnancy, but you should feel more settled by the second trimester.

I'm fine one minute and in tears the next. Is this normal?

Yes, it's quite common to have major fluctuations in your emotions during pregnancy. The hormones progesterone and oestrogen are thought to be partly responsible, but much of your moodiness is simply due to the fact that pregnancy is a time of tremendous change. You may be overjoyed at the thought of having a baby one day, then just as quickly begin wondering what it is you've got yourself into. Even when a baby is very much wanted, many ecstatic mothers-to-be find that concerns about the future momentarily cloud their happiness. You may be worried about how your relationship will be affected, the health of the baby you're carrying, and how you'll handle future financial challenges. Some of the minor problems of pregnancy, such as heartburn, fatigue and frequent urination can also be a burden. All these concerns may take your emotions on a roller-coaster ride.

I really hate feeling down. How can I manage my mood swings?

Mood swings are part of the pregnancy experience. It's not surprising that you're feeling highs and lows, sometimes from one minute to the next. Knowing that you're behaving as expected (and as your hormones dictate) may reduce some of the guilt you may be feeling. If you're down in the dumps, do something that makes you feel good. Take a nap, go for a walk or see a film with a friend. Don't be too hard on yourself. One of the best antidotes is talk therapy – literally.

Talk through your feelings with your partner, friends and family or, if you prefer, with your doctor or midwife. Pregnancy is a life-changing event, one

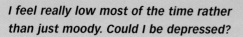

ASK THE EXPERT
ANNA MCGRAIL
BABYCENTRE EXECUTIVE EDITOR

I feel really low most of the time rather than just moody. Could I be depressed?

Yes, it's possible. Healthcare professionals sometimes don't recognize depression in pregnant women because they're conditioned, like the rest of us, to believe that this is a time of joy. Because we live in a society that expects pregnant women to glow and be happy, we tend to gloss over any sadness or depression, chalking it up to the usual moodiness that comes with pregnancy. Unfortunately, if overlooked, depression during pregnancy can hamper a woman's ability to care for herself and her developing baby.

You may be suffering from depression if you experience four or more of the following symptoms for a period of at least two weeks: anxiety, extreme irritability, sleep problems, exhausting or unending fatigue, a desire to eat all the time or not wanting to eat at all. A sense that nothing feels enjoyable or fun, persistent sadness, and frequent mood swings are also signs of depression. If this sounds like you, talk to your doctor or midwife about how you feel.

that's bound to make anyone – even someone who has wanted a baby for years – sometimes feel overwhelmed, irritable and anxious.

Am I going to have these emotional ups and downs throughout my pregnancy?

Mood swings tend to be most pronounced in the first 12 weeks of pregnancy. They should gradually diminish as you adjust and as your body adapts to the hormonal onslaught. It's normal to start feeling better and a bit calmer in the second trimester, but you might experience further ups and downs in the final weeks (pp 148–9).

I really can't seem to shake off my moodiness. What should I do?

If you feel like your mood swings are more than run-of-the-mill, it may be a good idea for you to see a counsellor. About 10 per cent of expectant women battle mild to moderate depression throughout pregnancy (see left). If you often or consistently feel blue, you may fall into this category.

I've suffered from depression in the past. If I get depressed during pregnancy, will it harm my baby?

Research suggests that when you're depressed, your body generates chemicals like the stress hormone cortisol, which can have an adverse effect on your baby. What's more, extreme stress is linked to a higher rate of miscarriage and premature birth. Also, being depressed may get in the way of you taking proper care of yourself while you are pregnant, in terms of eating properly, getting plenty of rest, avoiding drugs and alcohol and getting proper antenatal care. If you think you might be suffering from depression at any stage of your pregnancy, speak to your doctor.

JUST FOR DAD
Handling your partner's moods
The mood swings many women experience during pregnancy can leave the men in their life feeling very confused.

The causes: Understanding how women feel and behave when they're pregnant can be a challenge! Every woman is different, but all women are affected by hormonal, emotional and, obviously, physical changes during pregnancy. These changes can affect their mood from one moment to the next in ways they don't always understand themselves.

What you can do: Just showing that you understand your partner's moods could make all the difference to how she feels. You could ask if there's anything you could do to help (it's better to ask her when she's in a good mood as you're more likely to get an honest reply). You could also ask her to help you learn about pregnancy, too – she'll be pleased to know that you're interested, and it will help you to be more understanding when she does get moody. Stay informed by going to antenatal classes, reading pregnancy books and talking to other dads.

BabyCentre Buzz

"Listening to the experiences of other pregnant women helps me. It's reassuring to know that this feeling is a normal part of pregnancy and I'm not the only one with ups and downs." Melissa

"When I have a bad day, I write down all the positive things that are happening in my pregnancy, how excited we are about the little one's arrival, and then I sort of 'talk' to the baby. It gives me a sense of hope and excitement about what's to come and makes me feel better." Annabel

"My moods and emotions become hard to handle when I haven't had enough rest and I'm eating badly. When I feel down, taking my dog for a walk seems to help." Emily

"I find that buying something to do with the baby or maternity wear each week really picks me up." Joanne

Anxiety is spoiling my pregnancy. What can I do?

For some women the joy of finding out they're pregnant is quickly replaced by anxiety. The first trimester, in particular, is a time of unknowns – you may not have had any antenatal checks yet and, if you're not showing, may even wonder if you are actually pregnant. Take one day at a time and share any concerns with those close to you.

I've been very anxious since finding out I'm pregnant. Is this normal?

Pregnancy brings out the worrier in all of us. And for good reason: you're growing a life inside of you. It's natural to be concerned about what you eat, drink, think, feel and do. It's also perfectly normal – provided you don't obsess about it – to worry about whether your baby is healthy, to wonder how this new person will change your life and relationships, and to fret about whether you're truly up to the task of parenthood. However, if your anxiety is becoming all-consuming and regularly interferes with your day-to-day functioning, you need to find ways to relax and keep things in perspective.

I'm pregnant, but am worried I'll miscarry again. How can I calm down?

Try to remember that this pregnancy is different. While you may find yourself reflecting on what might have been, it's important that you also look forward to your future baby. Some women feel they can't really believe in the new pregnancy – but once they pass the point of the previous loss, they start to feel more positive.

It may well be that you're feeling anxious much of the time. But as you reach each milestone, such as hearing your baby's heartbeat or feeling the first movements, you'll feel more and more confident about the pregnancy. Having regular antenatal check-ups can also reassure you that your baby is doing well. Ask to see a midwife between appointments to listen to your baby's heartbeat if it makes you feel better. Try to take things one day at

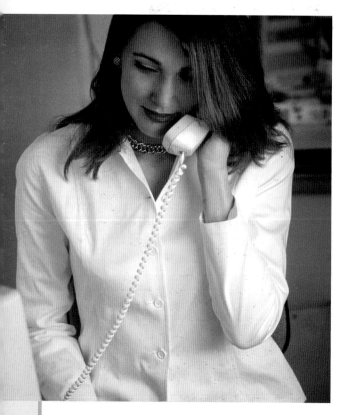

SEEKING ADVICE If you find that you're worrying about any aspect of your pregnancy, phone your doctor or midwife. They will probably be able to put your mind at rest.

a time. Easier said than done, but it can really work. When you feel yourself worrying, stop yourself and think only about today. It can also help to find out what happened last time. If a past loss was caused by cervical weakness, for example, read as much as you can about that condition. You may feel more in control of your situation if you understand what happened before. Unfortunately, many miscarriages and stillbirths don't have explanations. But the good news is that a past miscarriage, or even two, only increases the risk of having another one in the future very slightly. The vast majority of women who have lost a baby go on to have completely normal, healthy pregnancies.

Should I share my fears with my partner or will I just end up worrying him too?

Yes, do talk to your partner because the chances are he has concerns of his own. Talking openly about your anxiety can help you both feel better. You can also turn to friends or family members for support. Other mums-to-be are often a great source of comfort, too, as they're likely to be experiencing

the same worries. If you're extremely anxious or have a specific reason to be concerned about your baby's health, talk to your midwife.

I'm worried about my first scan and tests. Is this normal?

Anticipating the procedures, then awaiting the results, is a guarantee of some anxiety. Chances are that everything will be fine, so try not to fear the worst. Take it one step at a time. If something does come up, talk about your options with your midwife, and take time to think things through with your partner. Remind yourself that a positive result for a screening test doesn't necessarily mean there's a problem – it merely signals a need for more testing.

JUST FOR DAD

What you may be worried about

Security fears: The biggest fear men face is one deeply ingrained in our culture: will I be able to protect and provide for my family? When a baby arrives, there's often a temporary shift from two incomes for two people to one income for three. And that's a tough burden to carry. Plus, you have to be strong in ways you hadn't counted on before. You have to provide support not just financially but also emotionally. Your partner will need your help; and you have to be ready for her to lean on you.

Paternity fears: It's common to question – ever so fleetingly – how this baby can really be yours. It's not that you mistrust your partner's fidelity; it's just that you're momentarily overwhelmed by the idea that you had a hand in creating something as miraculous as a child.

Mortality fears: When you're a part of the beginning of a new life, you can't avoid thinking about the end of life. Thoughts about your own mortality can loom large: you're not the young buck any more, the next generation is in the works, and if everything turns out the way it's supposed to, you'll die before your child does. For a lot of young men who go around thinking they're immortal or invincible, that's a lot to absorb.

We planned this baby together, so why don't we feel the same now?

Even when a pregnancy is planned, it can take time to get used to the idea that you're actually going to have a baby. Pregnancy may affect you and your partner differently; give each other time to adjust and keep the lines of communication open.

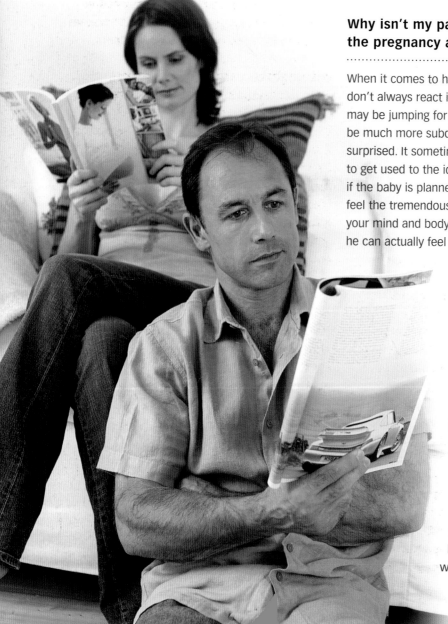

Why isn't my partner as excited about the pregnancy as I am?

When it comes to having a baby, men and women don't always react in the same way. While you may be jumping for joy, your partner's reaction may be much more subdued. If that's the case, don't be surprised. It sometimes takes a few months for men to get used to the idea of becoming a father, even if the baby is planned. Your partner can't yet see or feel the tremendous changes that are happening in your mind and body – so until you start to show or he can actually feel the baby kick when he puts his hand on your belly, your pregnancy may seem purely theoretical to him.

Your partner may also be worried about how your relationship (sexual and otherwise) is going to change once the baby is born, and whether he'll be a good father. Don't forget, too, that impending fatherhood often makes men feel under pressure to boost their earning power, get on the fast track at work and shoulder more responsibility in their daily lives. No wonder he's a little withdrawn and anxious!

BabyCentre Buzz

"Men are confusing: they send mixed signals and aren't always good at expressing their feelings. He may be overjoyed about the new baby, but he may also be afraid of what's to come." Carolyn

"Your partner may have deep worries about your health and how your relationship is going to change. Talk to him about your feelings and ask about his. Try not to condemn him for seeming unexcited at this point." Justine

"Don't let your partner's lack of enthusiasm dampen your spirits. Happiness is contagious. Find support from other family members and friends until he comes around." Jean

How can I get my partner to share his feelings about the pregnancy?

Many men keep their fears about pregnancy and fatherhood to themselves because they don't want to add to their partner's worries. Talk to him. Tell him you want to know how he's feeling and reassure him that he's not burdening you. Many men don't realize that women value this kind of interaction and that sharing their feelings will lead to greater intimacy. Encourage him to seek out other expectant fathers or male friends who already have children. Suggest that he reads a book or magazine article about becoming a father, and that he attends antenatal classes with you.

I'm not enjoying my pregnancy. Is there something wrong with me?

Everyone expects women to be ecstatically happy to be pregnant, but there are many reasons why you might not be. Maybe you don't feel emotionally ready to be a mother or are already stretched to the limits by other children or other commitments – especially if this pregnancy wasn't planned. On the other hand, perhaps you thought a baby was what you wanted, but now, faced with the reality of your situation, you're not so sure. For many women, simply feeling ill and tired from morning sickness and other symptoms can spoil the enjoyment and excitement but their feelings change once they reach the second trimester and start to feel well again. Having negative reactions to your pregnancy doesn't spell disaster, but do talk to your partner openly and honestly about your feelings to prevent the pregnancy driving a wedge between you.

I'm single and scared about going through pregnancy alone. What can I do?

Whether by choice or circumstance, more women than ever are going through pregnancy without a committed partner by their side. As a single mum you are likely to experience many of the usual pregnancy highs and lows, but may also be grappling with other problems, such as legal or financial worries, judgmental friends and family and possibly difficulties with the baby's father.

It's important to build a support network. Find out if there are antenatal classes for single mums-to-be – or at least women only (see pp 132–3). If you have the Internet, get online at BabyCentre.co.uk and 'chat' to other women who are in your situation. Above all, focus on taking good care of yourself so that you can take care of your baby.

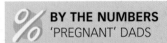

BY THE NUMBERS
'PREGNANT' DADS

Is her pregnancy making you look or feel like a different man?

26% *Yes, I think I am gaining more weight than she is.*

26% *No, I feel better than ever.*

23% *Yes, all the above apply.*

14% *Yes, I am pretty moody these days.*

11% *Yes, I feel a bit sick.*

Source: Based on a BabyCentre. co.uk poll of 486 dads-to-be.

When should we tell our family and friends?

Breaking the news to family and friends can be one of the most exciting aspects of pregnancy, especially if you've been keeping it a secret for weeks. You'll no doubt receive a positive reaction from most people, but accept that others, such as friends struggling with infertility, may find it difficult to share in your happiness.

I want to tell everyone I'm expecting a baby. Why do most women wait until 12 weeks to announce their pregnancy?

Some couples wait until they've passed the 12-week mark because the risk of having a miscarriage (see pp 18–19) drops significantly after this point. It means you're less likely to have to break sad news of a miscarriage to friends and family, which can be very difficult when you're already coping with your own feelings of loss.

Another reason some couples decide to wait is that they need time to get used to the fact they've conceived. It can take a while for concerns about becoming parents to surface, so this period is very useful for talking to each other and consolidating your thoughts and feelings about this new life-stage before telling everyone else.

BabyCentre Buzz

"I had to tell my family and friends because it was too hard to keep it a secret, but I managed to hide it from colleagues." Belinda

"We bought a bib that said 'Grandma loves me' and wrapped it up for my mother's birthday present." Diane

"I used crayons to write 'I'm going to be a big sister'. I took photos of my daughter holding it and emailed them to loved ones." Susmita

I'm dying to tell my best friend I'm pregnant. Is it wrong to do this when we've agreed to keep it quiet for now?

Try asking yourself how you would feel if your partner told his best friend. Would you feel let down, disappointed or angry? This would be because he'd acted in a way that goes against what you, as a couple, have planned to do. It might also make you think that his best friend is more important to him than you are.

Making joint decisions will form a crucial part of your relationship during the rest of your pregnancy and when you become parents. Agreements between couples are important as they're a way of establishing trust, which forms the basis of a good relationship. If you think telling your friend may damage the trust between you and your partner, think very carefully before you say anything.

My friend is having difficulty conceiving. How can I tell her I'm pregnant?

As you've sensitively recognized, your friend may be feeling vulnerable if she's having difficulty conceiving. But it's important you tell her about your pregnancy yourself rather than letting her hear about it from someone else. That could make her feel worse. Start your conversation by calmly and carefully acknowledging her position. Then be positive, tell her that you're pregnant and want her to know as she is a very good friend. She may struggle with this news, even shed a few tears, but if you can share her sadness with her and be supportive it may well reinforce your friendship.

My parents don't like my partner. Will they change their mind now I'm pregnant?

The excitement of becoming grand-parents may temporarily mask your parents' feelings of disapproval when it comes to your partner. They may be delighted and happy initially, but this may not be the case in the long term. Keep this at the back of your mind and try to see your pregnancy and the arrival of your baby as a time to work on your relationship with them. If, despite the news about your baby, they still make their disapproval obvious, you and your partner will need to work together to find ways of coping. Agreeing how often you will both see your parents can be helpful. Not responding to their negative comments will also show them your maturity and your commitment to your relationship.

My partner and I never wanted children, but now I'm pregnant I want the baby. How do I tell him?

It's best to tell your partner as soon as possible as you both have lots of thinking and talking to do. It may be that he's pleased about the baby, too. But if he's not, how will you both manage your relationship, given this life-changing event? If your relationship as a couple is a top priority then you'll probably both be fine. But if being childless is more important to him than your relationship, you may have to think about being a single parent.

How should we tell our teenage son we're having another baby?

When this kind of time-lapse pregnancy happens, parents can find themselves struggling to tell their older children. One reason is that it acknowledges your sexuality. It also means that family life, as your son has known it, is about to change dramatically.

If you think that your son is going through a vulnerable stage, reassure him that your feelings for him aren't going to change when the new baby arrives. However, most teenagers love having a baby in the family and enjoy their role as the older sibling in the family. If you and your partner are both pleased at the prospect of another family member, your teenager will almost certainly come to share your feelings in time.

How will my pregnancy affect our sex life?

While sex during pregnancy is almost always safe, actually wanting to do it – especially in the first trimester – may be the furthest thing from your mind. Try not to let a lack of intercourse become a problem between you and your partner, and remember there are other ways to maintain intimacy.

Can we have sex while I'm pregnant?

If your pregnancy is normal, you can continue to have sexual intercourse. However, there are reasons why some women may have to forego sex (see below) for a while. In any other circumstances, there is no physical reason why you and your partner cannot make love throughout pregnancy. If you have to hold off on intercourse for any reason, you can stay close through kisses, cuddles, massages and other ways of being affectionate.

JUST THE FACTS
RISK FACTORS

If you have any of the following conditions, ask your doctor what you can and can't do sexually, and at what point you should avoid sex:

- *Vaginal spotting or bleeding or unusual discharge.*
- *Abdominal cramping.*
- *Placenta praevia or a very low-lying placenta.*
- *Cervical weakness.*
- *Premature birth in a previous pregnancy or premature contractions in this pregnancy.*
- *Ruptured membranes (your waters have broken).*
- *An unhealed genital herpes lesion in either you or your partner, or the presence of any other untreated sexually transmitted infection.*

My partner thinks he'll harm the baby if we have sex. Is he right?

No. During intercourse, your partner's penis cannot damage the baby and you won't hurt the baby by making love, even with your partner on top. The mucus plug that seals the cervix helps guard against infection. The amniotic sac and strong muscles of the uterus also protect your baby. Though your baby may thrash around after orgasm, it's because of your pounding heart, not because he knows what's happening or feels pain. In later pregnancy, you may find it uncomfortable to have your partner on top, so experiment with other positions (see pp 152–3).

Will having sex feel the same while I am pregnant?

Not necessarily, but most of the changes you'll experience are positive. You may find that, finally free from worries about getting (or not getting) pregnant, you enjoy sex more. Increased vaginal moistness helps smoothe the way, and increased blood flow to your pelvic area causes genital engorgement and heightened pleasure. But the same engorgement may give you an uncomfortable feeling of fullness, and you may have mild and harmless abdominal cramps during or immediately after intercourse. Seek medical advice if the cramps are accompanied by bleeding. If your breasts are sore, your partner's caresses may feel painful.

JUST FOR DAD

Differences in desire

Changes in sexual desire – for you and your partner – are common during any time of major physical and emotional upheaval.

You: *For some men, pregnancy is an exciting confirmation of their masculinity and virility. In addition, a lot of dads-to-be feel closer to their partner than ever, and that closeness is often expressed erotically. So, at first, your partner's pregnancy might make you feel more sexy.*

For other men, the first trimester (and possibly the entire pregnancy) is a time of decreased desire. Before your partner got pregnant, she was the sexy woman you loved, and you probably thought about her body in a mainly sexual way. But now that she's pregnant, you may feel differently about her body – and think of it as more functional.

When her pregnancy's over, she's going to be a mother. And mothers aren't always seen as sexy. As the pregnancy progresses, these feelings may continue; a growing abdomen and leaking breasts in late pregnancy may seem more messy than enticing. Lots of men find their partner's growing body to be the essence of femininity and therefore attractive. Others don't.

Your partner: *A woman's feelings about sex can change from week to week or even day to day. Your partner may feel closer to you than ever and may be much less inhibited now that you don't have to worry about birth control. She may find the idea of having created a life with you to be wildly erotic, and she may be delighted with her blossoming body and new curves. On the other hand, she may be very tired and spend a lot of her first trimester hunched over the toilet in the grip of morning sickness – hardly an aphrodisiac.*

Finding solutions: *If you're as turned-on by your partner as ever – or even more so – tell her. She may want you just as much but be feeling insecure about her body right now. This is very common during pregnancy. You can put that anxiety to rest by being loving with or without intercourse. If she's giving you the cold shoulder, ask her why. Chances are, she simply feels too tired or too sick and may not realize that you're feeling rejected. Try not to take it personally.*

I don't always feel in the mood for having sex now that I'm pregnant. Is this normal?

Yes, absolutely normal. In the early months of pregnancy tiredness, nausea, breast tenderness and anxiety may mean that you don't feel like having sex very often. Don't feel bad about it – you're not going to feel like a tigress in the bedroom when your main goals are keeping your dinner down and staying awake beyond 8 pm.

My partner is still keen to have sex. How can I communicate my lack of interest without hurting his feelings.

Gently explain to your partner why you don't feel up to making love right now; ask him to be patient and reassure him that your lack of interest in sex doesn't mean that you love him any less than before. Both you and your partner should be reassured to know that your desire is likely to return when you're feeling better. In fact, you may find that making love in the second trimester (see pp 112–3) is better than ever. A man's libido may also be affected by pregnancy because he's concerned about harming the baby or because he has trouble adjusting to his partner's new shape (see left). While it is normal to go off sex, it's important for you and your partner to communicate so that it doesn't become a really big problem between you.

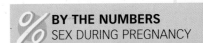

BY THE NUMBERS
SEX DURING PREGNANCY

How has pregnancy affected your sex life?

45% *Have sex less often than they used to.*

30% *Say they hardly ever have sex.*

13% *Say their sex life is pretty much the same.*

12% *Make love more often.*

Source: A BabyCenter.com poll of more than 52,000 people.

How will I cope at work?

Symptoms such as morning sickness and fatigue can wreak havoc on your workplace routine, especially if you're trying to keep your pregnancy a secret for now. You'll gradually devise some on-the-job coping strategies but, meanwhile, put yourself first and try to adapt your work and commuting routine as necessary.

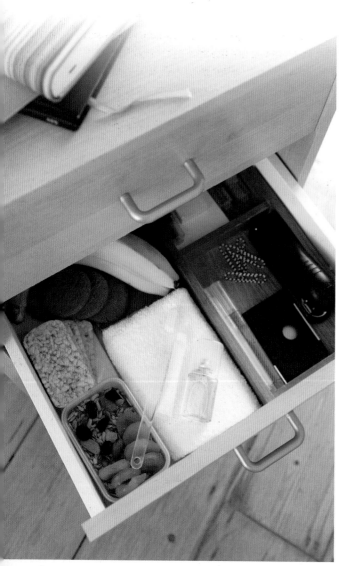

Is there any reason why I shouldn't work while I'm pregnant?

If you're having a low-risk, normal pregnancy and work in a safe environment, you can certainly continue working. UK Health and Safety regulations are in place to protect new and expectant mothers and their babies in the workplace, and employers are expected to be aware of, and if necessary remove, any risks or hazards that may affect you (see pp 116–17). If you feel that you are being exposed to any risk as a result of your employment (this could be because of the materials that you are exposed to, or having to do excessive travelling or shift work, for example), then you should talk to your Human Resources department.

What can I do to manage morning sickness at work?

If you are prone to vomiting, rather than just feeling nauseous, keep toiletries such as toothpaste, a toothbrush and wipes in your desk drawer. Also keep snacks that you know help to alleviate the sickness. If you haven't told colleagues your news yet, you could come up with a few convincing lines about 'food poisoning'. However, you may find

RESCUE KIT If you're prone to vomiting, keep a hand towel and a toothbrush and toothpaste or mouthwash in your desk drawer or handbag. Have snacks to hand, such as ginger biscuits, that you know will help to ease any queasiness.

BabyCentre Buzz

"Getting as much rest as I can prior to a big day of meetings helps me cope with those midday yawns." Helen

"I 'disappear' into an unused conference room, then lay my head down and have a quick catnap. One of my colleagues keeps an eye on the clock and comes to wake me after 20 minutes. Of course, you need sympathetic friends and an accommodating work environment to pull this off!" Holly

"If you have a safe place to park, take a nap in your car at lunchtime. Just make sure someone knows where you are and can wake you up!" Emma

that they put two and two together as they gather evidence that points towards your pregnancy, such as lengthy periods in the toilet or your sudden disinterest in alcohol at work social gatherings. If you are suffering particularly severe and prolonged morning sickness, you may have to tell your boss about your pregnancy earlier than planned.

How can I remain professional as my pregnancy progresses?

During the first and third trimesters, you may experience tiredness, absent-mindedness and daydreaming; during the second, you will probably feel more energetic and focused. It may help you to talk to a colleague who knows how it feels and can support you. There is likely to be a lot of interest in your pregnancy from colleagues as well as friends. Some women welcome this, enjoying the opportunity to talk about their growing baby. Others prefer their pregnancy to be part of their personal life, and not for discussion at work. You may have to be a little tolerant at first if people want to discuss it more than you would like. Remember, too, that

the novelty of the pregnancy will soon wear off for your colleagues and interest will diminish very quickly. Fortunately, it is now easy to buy business maternity wear, so you can continue to look smart and professional at work, even as your pregnancy reaches its final stages.

My work involves a lot of travelling and moving of equipment. Should I avoid this now that I'm pregnant?

You are legally protected from working with risks that could affect the health and safety of you or your unborn baby. Employers of women of childbearing age must carry out an assessment of any health and safety risks their employees and others could be exposed to. Lifting of heavy loads and travelling during the course of your employment are working conditions that may affect your health during pregnancy and so should be part of a risk assessment (see pp 116–17).

Your employer should do all that is reasonable to remove or reduce any risks, which could include altering your working conditions, offering you a suitable alternative, or suspending you on full pay if no alternative is available. If you are worried, talk to your doctor or get in touch with your local Health and Safety Executive office for advice.

IF YOU DO NOTHING ELSE...

- *If you sit at a desk all day, keep a box or stool underneath so that you can put your feet up.*
- *Take breaks. Stand up and stretch if you've been sitting for long periods; sit down and rest if you've been standing for long periods.*
- *Make your work space as comfortable as possible.*
- *Eat properly and avoid the workplace diet of constant coffee (or at least make sure there's decaf).*
- *Accept help when it's offered.*

When is the safest time to go on holiday?

It is safe to go on holiday during pregnancy provided you don't have any serious pregnancy complications. However, you'll find that most airlines won't take you during the final weeks. Most mums-to-be don't feel up to going away in the first trimester, but find that the second trimester is an ideal time to take a holiday.

Is it safe to fly during pregnancy?

Yes, although if you have pregnancy complications such as spotting, diabetes, high blood pressure or a previous premature delivery, check with your doctor before travelling. As long as your pregnancy is normal, it's safe to go ahead and make travel plans as usual. Most expectant mums find that the second trimester – weeks 14 to 27 – is a perfect time to travel. With morning sickness behind you, your energy levels high and the chances of miscarriage low, you can enjoy the luxury of relaxing, sleeping in and staying up late. You can also take advantage of the fact that you are still able to travel light – with no car seat, buggy, nappies or toys in tow. As long as you don't have medical complications, aren't expecting more than one baby and haven't had any prior premature deliveries, you can fly on most airlines until 36 weeks of pregnancy. Travel agents and airlines won't ask if you're pregnant when you book your seat, but you may be challenged at the check-in desk. For this reason, from about 28 weeks of pregnancy you will need a letter from your doctor confirming your due date and stating that you are unlikely to go into labour on the flight. Each airline has its own set of rules, so it's important you tell the booking agent when you call that you are pregnant and check that you may still fly (don't forget it applies to your return trip, too). If you are booking online, check the airline's website.

Will I be able to get travel insurance?

Because pregnant women are relatively high risk, many insurers stipulate they will not provide cover if the woman has less than eight weeks to go to her due date on the day she returns from holiday (around 32 weeks pregnant for most women). Other insurers have an even lower threshold of 27 or 28 weeks. That means that while you could still claim for losses unrelated to your pregnancy, you would not be covered if you had to cancel your holiday or incurred losses in connection with your pregnancy. If you are used to travelling frequently and already have an annual policy, you will need to call your insurer for advice on its rules. If not, you can shop around for a single policy, remembering to tell insurance providers you are pregnant.

What sort of holiday should I choose?

Opt for comfort over adventure, a degree of civilization and a reasonable standard of hygiene and medical care. Choose shortish flights that are

QUICK TIP

A European Health Insurance Card (EHIC) allows you free or reduced-cost medical care. It is not a substitute for travel insurance as it only covers emergency care. It is valid for three to five years and should be kept with you at all times.

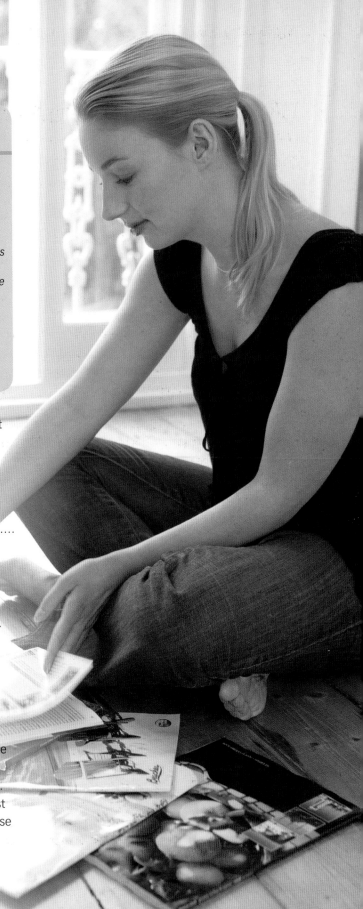

north–south rather than east–west to minimize jet lag and look for places where the temperature will be pleasant rather than boiling hot.

Is it safe to have travel vaccinations during pregnancy?

Most experts would advise against having vaccinations during pregnancy if they can be avoided. Before booking an exotic holiday, check what vaccinations, if any, are needed. It's important to balance the benefits against the risk. If you can choose a different holiday destination where no vaccinations are needed then it makes sense to do that. If you are staying in high-quality accommodation with good water supplies for two weeks, the risk factors will be low. If you are backpacking and living in rural areas for a month or two, the risk factors will be higher. Some people have to work in countries where there is a risk of a disease, or need to visit relatives who live there. In this case, talk to your doctor, or visit a specialist travel clinic to discuss the likely risks of the disease against the possible risks of the vaccination.

How will we manage financially?

Having a baby may trigger financial concerns for you and your partner, especially if you want to extend your maternity leave or give up work altogether. It's a good idea to review your income and outgoings to work out where you can make savings, and find out about any benefits you may be entitled to.

I'm worried that we're not going to have enough money once our baby arrives. How can we start making savings?

Few people have any idea what they spend on a weekly, monthly or annual basis. And most are shocked when shown in black and white their sheer waste of hard-earned cash on frivolities and useless consumer goods. If you want to cut down, the best way is to write down everything you spend for a month and analyze it. You'll probably feel better if you get rid of the dissatisfying spending: the items you buy and never use, or those you feel guilty about. It's also possible to cut 15 to 25 per cent from your outgoings with a few simple steps.

Start by reviewing your mortgage, credit cards, insurance and utility accounts. There are some very good deals around and you may be paying too much; by switching companies you should keep pace with the best deals around. Get rid of your overdraft facility and credit and store cards to reduce the temptation to use them. That way you'll never be able to buy things for which you don't have the money. If you really can't bear to get rid of your credit cards, shop around for one that has a lower interest rate or allows free balance transfers.

Should I save first or start to pay off my debts?

You should pay off debts as quickly as possible, because the interest rate you're paying on the debt is bound to be greater than the interest rate you would earn from your savings. Financial advisors say that the only 'good debt' is mortgage debt. Make sure you know the details of all your loans, credit and store cards. You should start by reducing your most costly debts first, especially your credit cards. These tend to have the highest interest rates or incur late-payment fees. However, be aware that for some forms of credit you can be penalized for paying in advance, so read the small print.

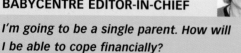

ASK THE EXPERT
DAPHNE METLAND
BABYCENTRE EDITOR-IN-CHIEF

I'm going to be a single parent. How will I be able to cope financially?

If you don't work or you work less than 16 hours a week, you may well qualify for Income Support or income-based Job Seekers' Allowance (JSA) plus Housing Benefit. You may be entitled to free milk and vitamins for yourself while you're pregnant and for your baby until he's five – ask at your doctor's surgery. You may also get money towards the cost of trips to and from hospital for antenatal and postnatal care. If you're on Income Support or the JSA, or you qualify for full Child Tax Credit, you should also qualify for Council Tax Benefit, plus a Sure Start Maternity Grant to buy clothes and equipment for your baby. If you work 16 or more hours a week, you may be eligible for the Working Tax Credit. For more information, contact your local Job Centre Plus or Social Security office.

I'm 12 weeks pregnant. Should I start saving now?

Yes, save as much as possible before your baby is born, regardless of your future plans. It's sensible advice for everyone to have three months' emergency money and if you haven't got it already now is a good time to build it up. Chances are you'll be too tired to go out and may not feel like buying new clothes, so use your surplus income wisely.

I know I should be saving, but what if I can't bear budgeting?

Don't say budget, say spending plan. Budget is one of those self-deprivation words like diet that only the truly masochistic can stick to, whereas a spending plan is about prioritizing to get the things you want. Write down everything you spend for a few weeks to see where you waste money. For example, do you eat out twice a week? Or do you drive to the shops when you could push the pram, saving petrol and parking charges? Organize your spending into fixed, variable and discretionary, and then prioritize each item.

How do I find out what benefits I'm entitled to?

You should be able to find useful literature and forms for the various benefits at your local post office, and possibly at your doctor's surgery or hospital clinic. The most useful document is the BC1 Babies and Children leaflet. The Department of Health's Birth to Five booklet is also helpful – you should be able to get this from your midwife or health visitor.

You can also download any forms you may need to claim benefits online from the Department of Work and Pensions, Inland Revenue and Child Support Agency websites.

I've been told my baby will receive a Child Trust Fund payment. What is it?

The Child Trust Fund is a long-term savings and investment account for all children who were born on or after 1 September 2002. Every child who was born on or after this date is eligible to receive a voucher worth at least £250 from the government. If your family has a low income and receives the full amount of Child Tax Credit, your child will receive £500. The account belongs to the child and can't be touched until he or she turns 18.

Neither you nor your child will pay tax on any income or interest made from the account. Parents and relatives will be able to save up to another £1,200 a year into this fund tax-free if they wish. The government will make a further contribution to the account when your child is seven. The money is paid in the form of a voucher, which can then be used to open an account.

I want to give up work once I've had my baby, but how will my partner and I cope on one income?

Few double-income families can envisage losing an income, but women who decide not to return to work often find it financially easier than anticipated. There are costs associated with going to work, such as travel costs, buying lunches and coffees, buying more clothes and socializing with colleagues. You'll be amazed at how much can actually be saved once you aren't working.

QUICK TIP

Free dental care and free prescriptions are available to all mothers-to-be and new mothers (of babies up to a year old), regardless of their income. Ask your midwife for an exemption from payment certificate at your booking appointment (see p 32).

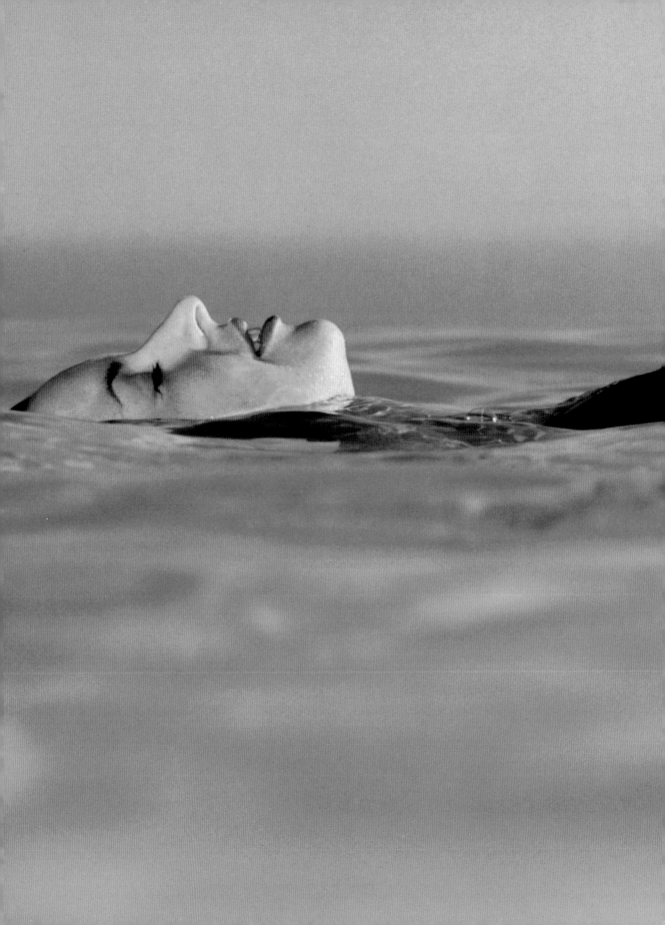

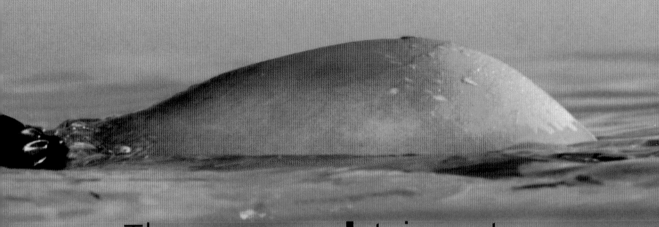

The **second** trimester

14–27 weeks

Like many women, you may begin to really enjoy your pregnancy this trimester. You're likely to be over the worst of the early symptoms, such as morning sickness, and be turning your attention to other important issues, such as what to wear! You can also unburden yourself of your 'secret' and share your exciting news with family, friends and colleagues.

14–27 weeks How will my baby develop?

During this trimester your baby will grow about 5 cm (2 in) each month. As she begins to stretch out, she will become much more active and even develop a range of facial expressions. By the end of this trimester all the major organs will be working, but her lungs and digestive system still won't be fully developed.

Your baby at 20 weeks

Around this time you may begin to feel your baby move and even get an occasional punch or kick. Her legs are gradually beginning to stretch out more now, instead of being curled up against her torso. As she moves and stretches, she's swallowing amniotic fluid, urinating and processing waste in her developing digestive system. She's producing meconium, a black, sticky by-product of digestion that accumulates in her bowels. You will probably see this meconium in her first nappy, although some babies pass it in the uterus or during delivery.

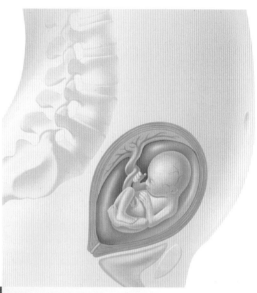

Your active baby

Your baby will become much more active and flexible this trimester and have far greater control because her muscles and nervous system are more developed. By around week 15, your baby will probably be able to grasp, squint, frown, grimace and maybe even begin to suck her thumb. Researchers believe these and other movements probably correspond to the development of impulses in the brain.

Week 14

Your uterus may be big enough by now to show the world that you're expecting, but your baby is still tiny. She's around 7–10 cm (3–4 in) long from crown to rump and weighs about 28 g (1 oz) – about the size of half a banana. Her unique fingerprints are already in place.

When you poke your stomach gently and she feels it, your baby will start rooting – that is, acting as if she's searching for a nipple. If you're carrying a girl, she already has approximately two million eggs in her ovaries, but she will only have a million by the time she is born.

Week 15

Your baby's body is now growing faster than the head. Around this stage of pregnancy, her parchment-thin skin covers itself with lanugo (ultra-fine, downy hair that usually disappears before birth). Your baby's eyebrows are beginning to grow and the hair on top of her head is sprouting.

Week 16

Your baby is still small enough to fit into the palm of your hand. There are new developments this week – light-sensitivity and a bad case of the hiccups, a precursor to breathing. You can't hear them because her system is filled with fluid rather than air, but don't be surprised if you feel them later on. Legs are growing longer than the arms now, fingernails are fully formed, and all the joints and limbs can move.

Week 17

Your baby is now about the size of an avocado, about 12.7 cm (5 in) long from crown to rump and weighs approximately 170 g (6 oz). During the next three weeks she'll go through a tremendous growth spurt, doubling her weight and growing in length by the day. Some of your baby's more advanced body systems are working now, including her circulation and urinary tract.

Babies are playful creatures, even at this stage. Yours may already have discovered her first toy – the umbilical cord – which she'll enjoy pulling and grabbing. Sometimes she may even clutch it so tight that less oxygen gets through, but don't worry – she doesn't hold on to it long enough to harm herself.

Week 18

The rubbery cartilage that will become your baby's skeleton is about to start hardening into bone. A protective covering of myelin is beginning to form around her nerves, a process that will continue for a year after she is born. With the help of an electronic device, known as a Sonicaid, your baby's heartbeat can now be heard. There's nothing more comforting or exciting than hearing your baby's heartbeat galloping along. On days when you're worried about how your pregnancy is progressing, hearing the heartbeat lets you know that your baby is developing and growing.

Week 19

This week, you officially begin your fifth month of pregnancy. Your baby is able to both feel and hear. Admittedly at this stage all she can hear is your heartbeat and the flow of your digestive system, but soon she'll be able to detect noise outside the uterus and identify your voice.

If you have an ultrasound scan (see pp 38–9) at this time, you may be able to see your baby kick, flex, reach, roll or even suck her thumb. If you're having a girl, the vagina, uterus and fallopian tubes are in place. If it's a boy, the genitals are distinct and recognizable.

JUST THE FACTS
YOUR BABY'S SECOND TRIMESTER HIGHLIGHTS

During this trimester, your baby will:
- *Become more active and flexible.*
- *Possibly begin sucking her thumb.*
- *Be able to hear your voice.*
- *Begin to open her eyes.*

- *Reveal the organs that tell you whether it's a boy or a girl!*
- *Develop a covering of hair, called lanugo.*
- *Start growing bone to replace cartilage.*

Your baby at 24 weeks

As you might have realized from your own expanding middle, your baby is in major growth spurt mode. At just over 450 g (1 lb), she is still relatively lean for her frame, but she'll soon add more body fat to balance out her rapidly growing brain, limbs and lungs. Her skin is still thin and translucent at this stage, but that will start to change soon. Her lungs are developing 'branches' of the respiratory 'tree' as well as cells that will produce surfactant, a substance that will help her air sacs inflate once she is born.

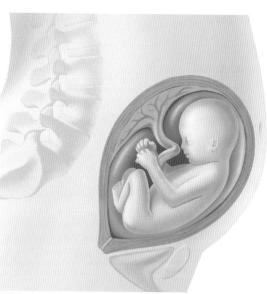

Lanugo

It's during the second trimester that your baby's body becomes covered by an ultra-fine covering of hair, called lanugo. This can appear as early as the 15th week of pregnancy. The first hairs usually grow around the baby's eyebrows and on the upper lip. Lanugo typically begins to disappear before the birth, and any that remains is naturally shed in the first few days. It will be replaced by hair that grows out of new hair follicles.

Week 20

Congratulations – you've made it to the halfway mark! Your baby is around 20.5 cm (8 in) long and weighs about 255 g (9 oz). She has started to swallow amniotic fluid, and her kidneys continue to make urine. Hair on the scalp is sprouting. Sensory development reaches its peak this week. The nerve cells serving each of the senses – taste, smell, hearing, sight and touch – are now developing in their specialized areas of the brain.

Week 21

Your baby is putting on weight now and has turned into a slippery little thing – a greasy white substance called vernix caseosa coats the entire body to protect the skin during its long submersion in amniotic fluid. Some babies are still covered with this whitish goo when they're born.

Week 22

Your baby's eyebrows and eyelids are fully developed and her fingernails now cover her fingertips. Watch what you say from now on because she will probably hear you! You can communicate by talking, singing or reading to her. Some studies suggest a newborn baby will suck more vigorously when breastfeeding if you read from a book she frequently heard during the time she was in the uterus.

Week 23

Your baby's lips are becoming more distinct and her eyes have developed; though the iris still lacks pigment for a few weeks yet. Her pancreas, essential for hormone production, is developing and the first signs of teeth are showing beneath her gum line.

Week 24

Your unborn baby probably measures about 30 cm (12 in). Blood vessels in her lungs are developing in preparation for breathing and she's swallowing amniotic fluid regularly, though she won't normally pass a motion until after birth. If your baby were to be born now, she would have a good chance of survival with the right care and thanks to the advances in science and technology.

Week 25

Your baby's gained about 115 g (4 oz) since last week. Her skin is thin and fragile but her body is filling out and taking up more room in your uterus. She is also starting to store up a layer of 'brown fat' in her chest, neck and groin. This helps to maintain her body heat.

Week 26

Your baby's beginning to make some breathing movements, though there's no air in her lungs as yet. Her senses are developing fast. At 26 weeks, fetal brain scans show that babies respond to touch and if you shine a light on your abdomen, your baby will turn her head. According to research, this shows that the optic nerve is functioning.

Week 27

Your baby measures about 37.5 cm (15 in) long with feet extended. If you could see your baby now, you might be able to get a glimpse of her eyes, which are now beginning to open. Response to sound grows more consistent toward the end of the sixth month, when the nerve pathways to the ears are complete. She also continues to take small breaths and, although she's only breathing in water and not air, it's good practice for when she's born.

14–27 weeks How will my body change this trimester?

You're officially in your second trimester. That's great news for two reasons. Firstly, your risk of miscarriage has dropped dramatically, and secondly, many women see early pregnancy symptoms, such as morning sickness, subside.

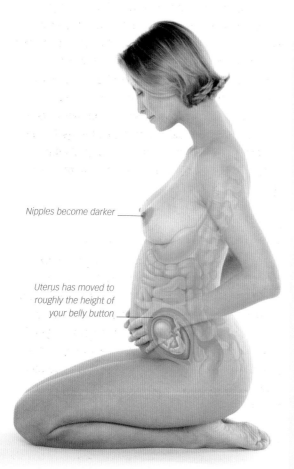

Nipples become darker ____

Uterus has moved to roughly the height of your belly button ____

GROWTH OF THE UTERUS *Your uterus has grown well into your abdomen – the top of it probably reaches your belly button. From now on it will grow at about 1 cm (0.4 in) per week. You may also notice some aching in your lower abdomen. It's nothing to be alarmed about – it's just the stretching of the muscles and ligaments that are supporting your bump.*

Your body at 20 weeks

You are halfway to the finish line, and you'll find that your body is ripening by the minute. Not only is your belly in full bloom, but – thanks to increased pigment levels – your nipples are a deeper hue. The normally invisible line that runs from your belly button to your pubic bone is darkening. This is known as the linea nigra (see p 96).

You can expect to gain around 450 g (1 lb) per week from now on. It's important to ensure you're eating a diet rich in iron (see p 98) to keep up with your expanding blood volume and to meet the needs of your growing baby and placenta.

Your immune system

During pregnancy the immune system can become slightly impaired so you may have more coughs and colds than normal. Although they are annoying and tiring, these sniffles won't harm your baby. Other infections such as chicken pox and rubella (see p 35) can cause problems for your baby depending on the stage of pregnancy when you catch them. However, most women have either had these infections already or, in the case of rubella, have been inoculated against it.

Week 14

You're probably feeling brighter and livelier than in the first three months now that you've put the early symptoms of pregnancy firmly behind you. Some unlucky women do find that the nausea drags on so if you are still being very sick, contact your midwife for advice. Birth is still months away, but your breasts may have already started making colostrum, the first milk that nourishes your baby immediately after birth, before the mature milk starts to flow.

Week 15

As you begin to feel more energetic, try some activities such as swimming, walking and low-impact aerobics. It's also a good time to sort out practicalities with your partner, such as assessing your finances, discussing your maternity leave and thinking about your childcare options (see pp 118–19), if you intend to return to work after your baby is born.

Week 16

Around this time you will be offered an antenatal blood test to screen for birth defects. The multiple marker screening test, which measures levels of alpha-fetoprotein (AFP) among other things, is usually performed between 15 and 20 weeks. You may also be offered the diagnostic test, amniocentesis, at this time (see p 86).

Week 17

You've probably gained at least 2.2 kg (5 lb) by now, and maybe as much as 4.5 kg (10 lb). Your uterus is growing and you might feel pangs caused by the ligaments stretching in your abdomen. These pains are usually temporary but your growing uterus will put extra strain on your back. It's a good time to arrange a last minute holiday if you can spare the time and money. Travelling in the middle trimester (see pp 120–1) is often recommended because you are usually over the early pregnancy feelings of nausea and fatigue and still not too far advanced for size or premature labour to be a problem.

Week 18

First-time mums often start to feel their baby's movements around now or in the next couple of weeks. Many women report that the first sensations are fluttery or like butterflies in the stomach. Unfortunately, your partner won't be able to share in your excitement just yet – real kicking doesn't usually start for a month or so. As your body gently expands, you may feel less than glamorous. Even if you don't feel attractive your partner probably still finds you a turn-on – many men find the rounder figure very appealing.

Week 19

You're just a week away from the halfway mark. In the next few weeks you'll probably have an ultrasound scan (see pp 38–9) to check your baby's organs. Seeing your baby curled up inside you is immensely moving so take your partner with you if you can. If your pregnancy is problem-free, you're unlikely to have anymore ultrasound scans so this may be your last opportunity to buy a scan photo for your baby's album.

Week 20

Getting a good night's sleep when you're pregnant can be difficult, particularly if you have heartburn or indigestion (see p 144). Adapt your diet to try to prevent these conditions and use pillows to support your bump (see p 94) so that you can get a better night's sleep.

JUST THE FACTS
YOUR SECOND TRIMESTER HIGHLIGHTS

During this trimester, you will:
- *Finally feel your baby's movements.*
- *Start to feel better as morning sickness and early pregnancy fatigue subside.*
- *Look better and possibly develop a 'glow'.*

- *Possibly develop new symptoms such as aches and pains and heartburn.*
- *Be offered blood screening tests and possibly a diagnostic test, such as amniocentesis.*

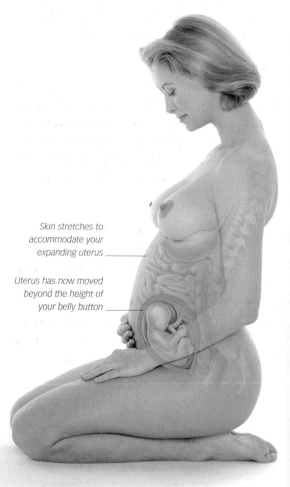

Skin stretches to accommodate your expanding uterus

Uterus has now moved beyond the height of your belly button

PRESSURE FROM THE UTERUS *As your uterus expands, it will begin to put pressure on the veins that return blood from your legs to your heart, as well as on the nerves leading from your trunk to your legs. This can lead to symptoms such as leg cramps (see p 92) and varicose veins (see p 137).*

Your body at 24 weeks

With your bump expanding by the day and your breasts increasing in size, you may have no choice but to invest in maternity wear, or simply adapt the clothes you have (see pp 108–9). The good news is that you've probably got that wonderful pregnancy glow (see p 96).

You may begin to notice more aches and pains, mainly in your lower abdomen and legs, and begin to suffer from fluid retention (see pp 92–3). Although early pregnancy fatigue will have passed, you may still feel tired from being unable to get good quality sleep at night. This may be caused by vivid dreams that are common in pregnancy and by an inability to get comfortable in bed (see pp 94–5).

Stretch marks

You may notice faint red streaks, known as striae or stretch marks, on your tummy, hips, buttocks and breasts. Lots of women have itchy skin on their bump as well – pregnancy hormones can make your skin drier and stretching over a growing bump doesn't help. Rubbing on creams may soothe the itching but it won't get rid of stretch marks and is unlikely to prevent them. Stretch marks are typical at this stage of pregnancy and will fade after you give birth.

Week 21

You may have noticed changes to your skin and hair (see pp 96–7). While many of these are positive, others such as acne can be unwelcome. Be diligent about washing with a gentle cleanser twice a day, but don't take any oral acne medications as some of these are hazardous in pregnancy.

Week 22

Just how much weight you will gain by the end of pregnancy may be preying on your mind and you may be battling with food cravings (see pp 100–1) and a much healthier appetite. Always eat when you are hungry but try to choose healthy snacks rather than reaching for the sweets and biscuits.

Doctors and midwives are much more relaxed about weight gain in pregnancy now. Take the same approach and give yourself a break. It's also best not to worry immediately about losing weight after you've had your baby as your body can take anything from a few months to a year to recover nutrients used up during pregnancy. Do seek advice from your midwife, however, if your weight is soaring or plummeting. Your midwife will usually check to see if your bump is measuring about right for your dates (see p 84).

Week 23

It's common in pregnancy to have an increased vaginal discharge as the result of increased blood flow in that part of the body. Needing to go to the toilet more than usual is another unwelcome side-effect of pregnancy.

You are also more susceptible to urinary tract infections, too. See your doctor or midwife if you suspect a bout of cystitis. You may also experience bleeding from your back passage, if you have developed piles (see p 145).

Week 24

You may notice some bleeding when you brush your teeth – a common pregnancy complaint (along with nosebleeds). Pregnancy hormones can make your gums swell and become inflamed, which leads to frequent bleeding, especially when you clean your teeth. Brush and floss regularly but gently. Although you may want to avoid disturbing your gums, it's crucial to practise good dental hygiene during pregnancy to avoid gum disease. Dental treatment is free while you are pregnant.

Week 25

You might want to start thinking about baby names if you haven't already. Choosing a name can be fun, but you may be surprised at how difficult it can be to reach a decision (see pp 106–7). There are plenty of baby name books and websites to help you.

Week 26

If you have a swab to check for a vaginal infection such as thrush, the results may come back positive for group B streptococcus too. This is a common infection, but it can be dangerous for newborn babies. If you are found to carry the infection, you will be given intravenous antibiotics during labour to prevent the infection passing to your baby.

Week 27

You're nearing the home stretch – the third trimester. Before you know it, you'll be cradling your baby in your arms. Around this time, you may see a slight increase in your blood pressure, which is usual. But if your weight suddenly shoots up, or your vision blurs, and your hands, feet and face swell dramatically, you may have pre-eclampsia (see p 135) and must seek urgent medical help.

How is my pregnancy monitored?

Your regular antenatal checks are an opportunity for your midwife to check your progress and your baby's development. She will record her findings on your maternity notes. If your midwife has any concerns, she may recommend further scans but this is usually a precaution and shouldn't be a cause for concern.

What is a personal maternity record?

When you book for maternity care, you will be given a personal maternity record, which is usually referred to as your 'notes'. You need to take these to all your antenatal appointments and give them to your midwife when you go into labour. Remember to take them with when you go on holiday. If you need medical care while you're away, they will provide invaluable information for the people treating you. Also, if you need to contact a health professional in an emergency, all the numbers are on the front of your record. Your record tells your midwife and doctor exactly how your pregnancy is progressing. Some of your notes will be in an abbreviated form (see box, right).

I've been told the fundal height is large. What does this mean?

The fundal height is the measurement from the upper edge of your pubic bone to the top of your uterus. The tape measurements (in centimetres) should equal the number of weeks that you are pregnant within two centimetres, but this measurement can vary depending on your size and shape. Some women expecting second or subsequent babies tend to measure slightly large for dates in their first and second trimesters, possibly due to the fact that their muscles have been weakened by a previous pregnancy. If you are big for your dates, it can also indicate twins, a uterine fibroid, a large baby or simply a mis-measurement. The most likely explanation is that

CHECKING YOUR PROGRESS As your pregnancy progresses, the size of your uterus will be checked with a tape measure. This will give an indication of how well your baby is growing.

everything is quite normal and that there is no need to worry, but an ultrasound scan might be recommended to investigate further.

What does 'small for dates' mean?

This means that your baby is smaller than expected for your stage of pregnancy. It may be caused by a lower amount of amniotic fluid around your baby, which would make you appear smaller even though your baby is the right size. Your height, shape and abdominal muscles can also affect the measurement, as can the fact that babies grow at slightly different rates and are measured against averages. Some babies appear small for a while and then have a growth spurt. However, 'small for dates' can also indicate a problem known as intrauterine growth restriction (IUGR), in which the placenta doesn't work as well as it should. In this case, an ultrasound scan (see pp 38–9) will probably be recommended to measure different parts of your baby and you may be re-scanned two or three weeks later to check your baby's growth. If there are concerns about your baby's size, rest is quite effective as it increases placental blood flow.

I'm expecting my second baby. Why am I having so few checks this time round?

This is probably because you had a straightforward pregnancy last time. Until recently, there was a set pattern for checks in pregnancy. You would see a midwife for the first time at about 12 weeks and have about 12–15 antenatal checks in all. Government guidelines now suggest that 10 checks the first time around and seven in subsequent pregnancies are enough, provided your pregnancy is uncomplicated. Your antenatal appointments will be tailored to your needs and you may find that, though your visits are fewer, they are longer. If problems develop, you will be seen more frequently.

JUST THE FACTS
UNDERSTANDING YOUR NOTES

Here are some of the common abbreviations:

Length of pregnancy: *24+3 (24 weeks and three days pregnant).*

Blood pressure: *120/70 (the lower figure should not be higher than 90).*

Urine: *PGO (whether your urine sample contains Protein, Glucose or anything else — Other).*

Presenting part or lie:
Cephalic (or ceph) *– Head down.*
Br *– Bottom down or breech.*
LOA *– Left occipitoanterior: the back of your baby's head is on your left side and towards the front of your tummy.*
ROA *– Right occipitoanterior: the back of your baby's head is on your right side and towards the front of your tummy.*
LOP *– Left occipitoposterior: the back of your baby's head is on your left side and towards the back of your tummy.*
ROP *– Right occipitoposterior: the back of your baby's head is on your right side and towards the back of your tummy.*

Heartbeat or activity:
FHH *– fetal heart heard.*
FHNH *– fetal heart not heard (probably because your baby is in an awkward position).*
FMF *– fetal movements felt.*
FMNF *– fetal movements not felt.*

IF YOU DO NOTHING ELSE...

- *Attend all your antenatal appointments.*
- *Write down questions to ask your midwife to get the best out of your antenatal care.*
- *Keep your maternity records safe and take them with you if you go on holiday.*

What tests will I have this trimester?

You will be offered blood tests to assess your risk of having a baby with chromosomal abnormalities, such as Down's syndrome. If the results of the blood test show that the risk is high, you will be offered optional diagnostic tests, such as amniocentesis, that can confirm the result.

Will I have screening tests this trimester?

Yes. There are blood tests carried out between 15–20 weeks of pregnancy that measure various 'markers' in your blood, such as hCG (human chorionic gonadotrophin) and AFP (alpha-fetoprotein). The levels of these markers can be an indication of whether you are carrying a baby with Down's syndrome. There are several variations of this test available: the double test measures two markers; the triple test three markers; and the quadruple test four markers. The double test detects about 59 per cent; and the quadruple

ASK THE EXPERT
CHRISSIE HAMMONDS
MIDWIFE SONOGRAPHER

I'm feeling confused about all the tests. Should I just have everything I'm offered?

No, you should find out as much information as you can first. The National Institute for Clinical Excellence (NICE) states that pregnant women must be given information about any screening or diagnostic tests they are offered. You should have the chance to talk to a midwife, doctor or screening counsellor until you are clear about what the tests can and can't tell you. You can, for example, decide not to have any tests at all or to have a screening test, but not a diagnostic test. Seek advice at the earliest opportunity and then go away and think about what you want to do. Take your time and have only the tests that are right for you.

about 75 per cent. Blood tests are more accurate in older women (because older women are more likely to have babies with Down's). Remember, even if your screening test shows a high risk, it doesn't necessarily mean your baby has Down's. It's only a risk factor. But you will need to decide whether to have amniocentesis, a diagnostic test, for confirmation.

What is amniocentesis?

Amniocentesis is a diagnostic test, which means it can tell you with almost complete certainty whether or not your baby has a chromosomal abnormality. It involves taking a sample of amniotic fluid and examining it to see whether your baby has any serious chromosomal abnormalities, such as Down's or other syndromes.

Will I be offered amniocentesis?

It depends. Some hospitals routinely offer amniocentesis to all pregnant women over the age of 35 because these women are at higher risk of having a baby with Down's syndrome. You will also be offered an amniocentesis if you have had a positive screening test (see above). Other women who might be offered amniocentesis are those who have – or whose partner has – a family history of certain birth defects, or who already have a child with a genetic abnormality. Many hospitals offer

CVS (see p 37) rather than amniocentesis. The main advantage of this test is that it can be performed earlier, at around 10–12 weeks.

When will I have an amniocentesis test?

Amniocentesis is usually performed between weeks 15–18, but it can be performed after this if problems are found. Amniocentesis before week 14 has been shown to carry a higher risk of miscarriage. From 15 weeks of pregnancy, there is enough amniotic fluid to make it easier to take an adequate sample without putting the baby at risk.

How is amniocentesis performed?

Using ultrasound for guidance, your doctor will identify a pocket of amniotic fluid a safe distance from your baby and the placenta. He or she will then insert a long, thin, hollow needle through your abdominal wall and into the fluid to withdraw a sample. You can choose to have your abdomen numbed first with a local anaesthetic.

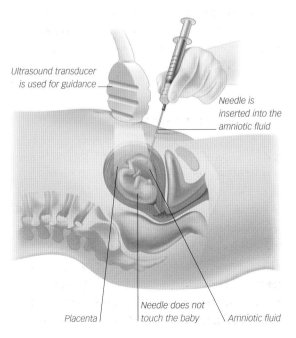

Ultrasound transducer is used for guidance

Needle is inserted into the amniotic fluid

Placenta *Needle does not touch the baby* *Amniotic fluid*

How long will it take for me to get the results of my amniocentesis test?

The sample of amniotic fluid has to be sent away to a laboratory to be cultured. It can take as long as 1–2 weeks to grow a sufficient number of your baby's cells to reach a diagnosis so you may have to wait 2–3 weeks. But in some areas the results may be available quicker.

The waiting period can seem very long indeed. You might find it helpful to have a full programme of activities during this time to keep yourself occupied. A new test called Amnio-PCR has been developed which can give results in 48 hours but this is only available privately.

What risks are associated with diagnostic tests and do they hurt?

About 1 in 100 women develops an infection or other complication that results in miscarriage. Some women leak amniotic fluid or lose a small amount of blood from the vagina. A high temperature, uterine contractions and/or tenderness, or feeling chilly and hot by turns indicate an infection. The risk of miscarriage is slightly higher (1–1.5 per cent) for chorionic villus sampling (see p 37) than for amniocentesis (0.5–1 per cent).

Diagnostic tests may be uncomfortable, and some women find them painful. However, the procedure lasts no longer than half an hour, and actually taking the sample lasts only a few minutes. Any stomach pains you experience afterwards will probably be minor, but a few women have serious cramps. Your midwife will advise you to rest for 24 hours as a precaution.

AMNIOCENTESIS *This specialized test involves taking a sample of amniotic fluid from the uterus, which is examined in the laboratory to check for chromosomal abnormalities. As well as detecting chromosomal abnormalities, amniocentesis can identify the sex of the baby and, in later pregnancy, whether the baby's lungs are mature.*

Is it normal to have aches and pains?

Most mid-pregnancy aches and pains are related to the extra work your body is doing to accommodate your growing baby. While some symptoms are barely noticeable, others can be very painful. Seek advice from your midwife or doctor about how to relieve any discomfort and, if necessary, you may be referred for physiotherapy.

My lower abdomen aches. Is this normal?

Yes, the aching is usually caused by the stretching of the muscles and ligaments supporting your uterus. You'll probably feel it when you're getting up from a seated position or when you cough. When you feel this aching, resting should alleviate your symptoms. Sit down, put your feet up and relax. Don't forget, it's a perfectly normal complaint of pregnancy, and it gives you an excuse to put your feet up and be waited on. Flexing your knees towards your abdomen may make you feel better,

or try lying down on your side with one pillow under your belly and another between your legs. Don't hesitate to call your doctor or midwife if abdominal aching is accompanied by severe pain, cramps, bleeding, fever, chills or a feeling of faintness.

Why do I often feel pain and numbness in my hands, and how can I relieve it?

Pain and numbness in your hands and fingers is most likely caused by carpal tunnel syndrome. The pain is usually centred in the thumb, index finger, middle finger and half of your ring finger. Symptoms can appear at any time but most commonly begin in the fifth or sixth month of pregnancy, along with mild swelling of the ankles and feet. It happens when swelling in the carpal tunnel in your wrist (the tube that the nerves going to your fingers run through) presses on the nerves. This pressure causes numbness, tingling, burning, and pain in the fingers and often up the arm.

If you get the symptoms at night, try wearing a wrist splint. This holds your wrist in position where the carpal tunnel is as 'open' as possible to relieve the pressure on the nerves. A doctor, midwife or physiotherapist will be able to give you one. Try flexing your fingers and hands regularly and, if possible, avoid jobs requiring repetitive hand movements as they can aggravate your symptoms. Sitting with your hands raised often helps, as can placing your wrists and hands in cool water.

ASK THE EXPERT
ALISON BOURNE
PHYSIOTHERAPIST

What is Symphysis Pubis Dysfunction (SPD), and how is it treated?

The two halves of your pelvis are connected at the front by a joint called the symphysis pubis. To help your baby's passage through your pelvis, a hormone is produced that softens the ligaments and causes the pelvic joints to move more than usual. Symptoms of SPD are pain in the pubic area and groin, a grinding or clicking in your pubic area and pain down the inside of your legs or between them. A pelvic support belt can provide relief. You may need physiotherapy on your hip, back or pelvis to correct any underlying problems and will be shown some useful exercises. You should be given advice on how to make daily activities less painful and on how to make the delivery easier.

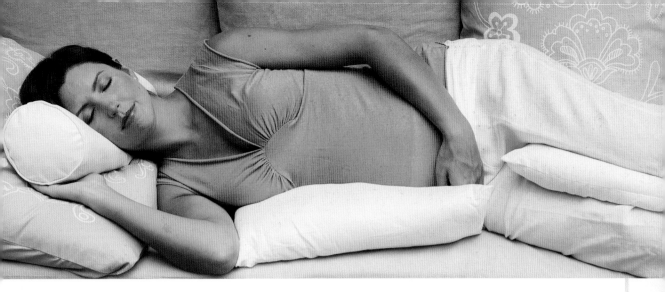

LOWER ABDOMINAL PAIN This common pregnancy complaint can be relieved by lying down and using pillows for support. Place one pillow under your bump and another between your legs.

Why are my hips sore?

The hormones released during pregnancy relax the ligaments supporting your joints. This happens almost from conception as nature's way of preparing the body for labour. The extra movement this allows around the joints of the hips and pelvis is helpful for giving birth. However, it can also lead to discomfort that might get worse as you increase in size and weight. Some people develop hip pain when their baby engages or moves down the pelvis.

How can I ease discomfort in my hips?

It is important to adopt a sleeping posture in which all the joints around the pelvis and hips are well supported, such as sleeping on your side with both legs bent and a pillow between the knees supporting the whole length of your leg. A pillow under your bump is also needed to stop you rolling forward. Putting an extra layer of padding, such as a sleeping bag or quilt, under your bottom sheet can also improve matters. You may also find gentle heat in the form of a hot water bottle on your hips helpful. Avoid sitting with your legs crossed, and to ensure you are sitting upright use a small, rolled-up cushion or towel to support the arch at the bottom of your back. You should also avoid activities which appear to aggravate the pain, too.
If the pain persists, seek medical advice

Is it safe to take painkillers?

Your choice of painkillers is more limited during pregnancy. Aspirin should be avoided as it has a blood-thinning effect, but low-dose aspirin may be prescribed if you've suffered recurrent miscarriage or have pre-eclampsia (see p 135). Ibuprofen isn't recommended as it may affect your baby and prolong labour. Paracetamol is considered safe at the recommended dose and only used occasionally. A study carried out at King's College, London and Bristol University found that mums-to-be who took paracetamol 'most days' or daily in late pregnancy were twice as likely to have a wheezy baby. Doctors recommend that pregnant women take it no more than 1–2 days per week. Avoid stronger painkillers that combine several ingredients and, if you suffer from migraines, seek advice from your doctor.

IF YOU DO NOTHING ELSE...

Seek medical advice if you have a severe or persistent headache and intense pain or tenderness in your upper abdomen. These are possible signs of pre-eclampsia (see p 135), a potentially serious condition.

Backache during pregnancy

Backache is a common complaint of pregnancy. Between 50 and 75 per cent of pregnant women get back or pelvic pain at some time. Although some back pain is inevitable, there are many ways to alleviate the discomfort and prevent it from turning into a long-term problem.

Causes of back pain

Backache during pregnancy can be caused by poor posture, injury or being 'out of condition' – the same as back pain in those people who are not pregnant. Most women with back pain in pregnancy, however, actually have something called Pelvic Girdle Pain. This is where the pelvic joints become looser or 'unlocked' because of softened ligaments. This type of pain is usually felt in the buttock area but can shoot down into the legs. It can sometimes be accompanied by pubic pain, just above the bladder.

Many doctors, midwives and physiotherapists don't know about Pelvic Girdle Pain, so it is important to see a physiotherapist with a qualification from the Association of Chartered Physiotherapists in Women's Health (see p 226). If you see a chiropractor or osteopath, make sure he or she is experienced in treating pregnant women.

A small percentage of women will suffer from sciatica during pregnancy. This is where pins and needles, pain and numbness in the leg is caused by inflammation or pressure on the sciatic nerve in the back. Pelvic Girdle Pain can sometimes be mistaken for sciatica.

Your posture

A good, upright posture can help with back and pelvic pain. If you slump or slouch, your pelvic joints can 'unlock' which causes pain. Make sure you stand tall and support your back with a cushion when you sit. Sitting on an upright chair with your back arched, your chest stuck out and your legs slightly apart will feel more comfortable than slouching on a sofa.

Protecting your back

Try the following to protect your back:
- Perform regular pelvic floor exercises (see p 105) and try to gently pull your belly button in and up at the same time. This helps to 'lock' your pelvic joints and control pain when you move. Being positioned on your hands and knees is a good way to try this exercise but you can also do it whilst sitting or standing.
- Studies have shown that you can reduce the risk of developing back pain (but not pelvic pain) if you exercise on a weekly basis. The most appropriate forms of exercise include swimming, walking, aquanatal classes, Pilates, yoga or cycling.
- If you have to lift or carry anything, hold it close to your body, bend your knees rather than your back (as if squatting) and try not to twist.
- If you have a toddler, see if they can climb onto a chair or sofa before you pick them up. Try to encourage more mobile children to climb into their car seats themselves.

USING A BIRTH BALL *Birth balls are great for encouraging good posture, easing aches and pains and exercising muscles. Try sitting on the ball and moving it backwards and forwards with your hips so that your back arches and 'slumps' in a rhythmical fashion. You can also move it from side to side or round in circles.*

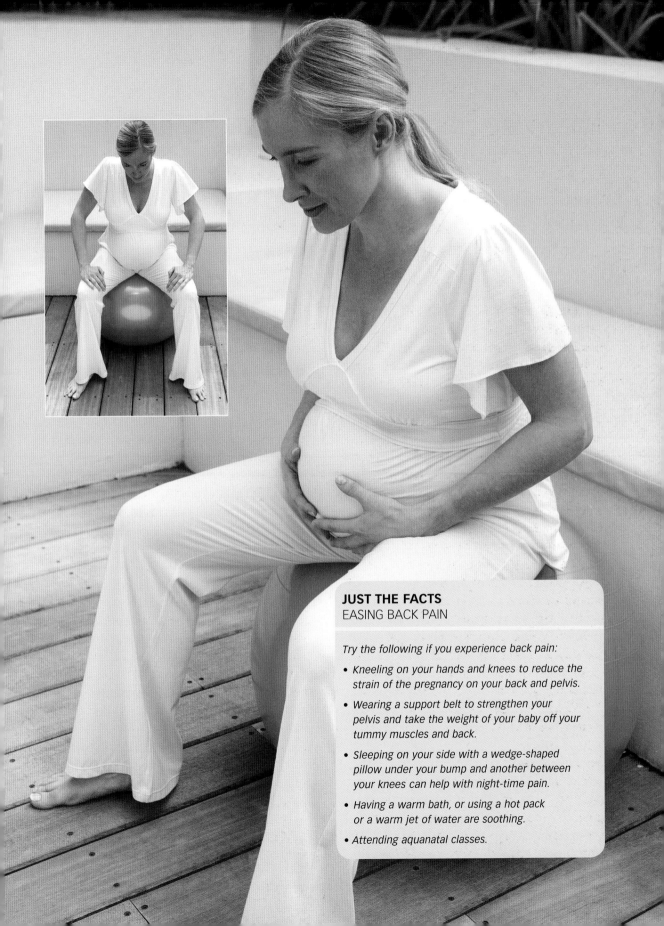

JUST THE FACTS
EASING BACK PAIN

Try the following if you experience back pain:

- *Kneeling on your hands and knees to reduce the strain of the pregnancy on your back and pelvis.*

- *Wearing a support belt to strengthen your pelvis and take the weight of your baby off your tummy muscles and back.*

- *Sleeping on your side with a wedge-shaped pillow under your bump and another between your knees can help with night-time pain.*

- *Having a warm bath, or using a hot pack or a warm jet of water are soothing.*

- *Attending aquanatal classes.*

I have leg cramps. Should I be worried?

Leg pains may start to plague you now and get worse as your pregnancy progresses. Sudden, sharp cramps sometimes strike during the day, but are most common during the night, disrupting sleep. Leg cramps are irritating, but not a serious condition, and it is worth trying different methods, such as changing your diet, to minimize them.

Why am I getting leg cramps at night?

The added weight on your leg muscles often leads to night cramps, which can wake you out of a sound sleep. Leg cramps hit hardest in the second and third trimesters. Some other possible causes are thought to be an excess of phosphorus (found in processed meats, snack foods and fizzy drinks) and a shortage of calcium circulating in your blood. The pressure of the expanding uterus on the nerves leading to your legs is also a factor.

Can I do anything to prevent cramp, and how can I relieve it?

Try stretching your calf muscles before going to bed and avoiding standing for long periods or sitting with your legs crossed. Get into the habit of rotating your ankles and wiggling your toes when sitting. Leg cramps can be caused by calcium deficiency so eat calcium-rich foods (see p 99). If you suffer badly with leg cramps, ask your midwife or doctor about taking a calcium supplement. Avoid consuming too many fizzy drinks, including so-called 'healthy' carbonated drinks that contain minerals and vitamins, as these contain a lot of phosphorus, which can sometimes exacerbate leg cramps.

When a cramp strikes, try stretching your leg immediately. Start by straightening your leg – heel first – and gingerly flexing your ankle and toes. This will hurt at first but gradually make the pain go away. Massaging the cramped muscle or walking it off can also help, as can taking a warm bath or placing a hot water bottle on the cramped area.

What if the pain persists?

If the pain is constant and not just an occasional cramp, or if you notice swelling or tenderness, call your doctor. You could have venous thrombosis, or a blood clot, a fairly rare but serious condition requiring immediate medical attention.

Should I be worried that my ankles and toes are swollen?

What you're experiencing is called oedema, which results from the extra blood you've acquired during your pregnancy. Your growing uterus puts pressure on your pelvic veins and your vena cava (a large vein on the right side of your body that receives blood from your lower limbs). This, plus the effects of pregnancy hormones, slows down your

QUICK TIP

To minimize fluid retention during pregnancy, make sure you drink plenty of water because, surprisingly, keeping hydrated helps your body retain less water. Exercise regularly and avoid eating salty foods, such as olives and salted nuts.

RELIEVING CRAMPS
If you get a cramp, immediately stretch your calf muscles: straighten your leg, heel first, and gently flex your toes back towards your shins. It might hurt at first, but the pain will gradually ease. You can also relax the cramp by massaging the muscle or warming it with a hot water bottle.

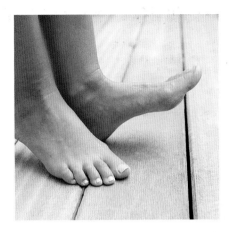
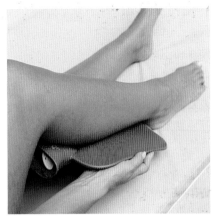

circulation and causes blood to pool in the lower half of your body. Pressure from the trapped blood forces fluid out into the tissues of your feet and ankles. Oedema is common and normal, but if you have severe swelling in your hands and face, seek medical advice: it could be a sign of pre-eclampsia (see p 135), a serious pregnancy-related condition.

How can I minimize the puffiness in my ankles and feet?

To control the oedema, raise your feet whenever possible. If you sit down all day long, it helps to keep a stool or pile of books under your desk; at home, sit with your feet raised or lie down preferably on your left side whenever possible. Putting on waist-high support tights before you get out of bed in the morning, so blood has no chance to pool around your ankles, will also help.

Restless leg syndrome is affecting my ability to sleep. What can I do?

Up to 15 per cent of pregnant women develop a condition called restless leg syndrome (RLS), when sensations in the feet and legs begin to disrupt sleep. Sufferers have an overpowering urge to move their legs and it usually gets worse later in the day

and at night. No one knows exactly what causes RLS and, while it is not considered a serious medical condition, its effects can range from mildly irritating to truly maddening.

Although there are several kinds of drugs to treat RLS, none can be taken in pregnancy. Try keeping a journal of your diet, activities and emotions. After a few weeks, you may be able to tell whether certain factors trigger RLS. You may find, however, that you have to live with this condition, at least until after your baby is born.

BabyCentre Buzz

"I don't know where I'd be without my clogs. It doesn't matter how wide my feet get, I can slip them on so easily – plus, I don't have to bend over to do up laces or a zip." Jocelyne

"I decided to invest in a pair of expensive but really comfortable walking shoes. I tried them on with extra-thick socks so if my feet get wider, they should still fit." Chloe

"Fortunately, I've been able to walk around in flip-flops all summer and haven't had to worry about squeezing into my winter shoes – yet." Anna

How can I get more sleep?

During this trimester you may have difficulty getting comfortable in bed and find that your sleep begins to be disrupted by strange pregnancy-related dreams. Although you're unlikely to be as tired as you were in the first trimester, it's still important to find ways of getting some good-quality sleep.

I'm finding it difficult to get comfortable in bed. What can I do?

Using pillows to support your belly and back can mean the difference between a sleepless night and a peaceful slumber. Regular pillows work fine, but you may want to invest in a pregnancy pillow: a wedge-shaped one supports your belly when you lie on your side. You can also use them to prop yourself up to a semi-reclining position when you're lying on your back. A full-length body pillow is a mega-pillow that is at least 1.5 m (5 ft) long and designed to support your back and cradle your belly. You can also buy a bean-shaped pillow that supports your belly and back, and this also makes a good nursing pillow later if you're breastfeeding.

Is it possible that my diet could be affecting the quality of my sleep?

Yes, what you eat and, more importantly, when you eat it, can affect the quality of your sleep. For example, drinking a glass of warm milk is known to aid sleep and some experts believe that foods high in carbohydrates, such as bread and pasta, can promote sleep, so make your late-night snack a carbohydrate-rich sandwich or a piece of toast. But if you suffer from heartburn (see pp 144-5) or restless leg syndrome (see p 93), you should choose another option because your symptoms may get worse if you fill up on carbohydrates.

If bad dreams, headaches or hot flushes are disturbing your sleep, the cause may be low blood sugar. Just before you go to bed, tuck into a high-protein snack, such as scrambled egg on toast or some beans on toast, to keep your blood sugar levels up during the night.

If you get hunger pains during the night, keep some healthy snacks on your bedside table to prevent you having to get out of bed, which can disturb your rest even further.

ASK THE EXPERT
DR MORAG MARTINDALE
GP

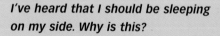

I've heard that I should be sleeping on my side. Why is this?

Once you get halfway through your pregnancy, it's wise to avoid sleeping on your back, a position that puts the full weight of your uterus on your spine, back muscles, intestines and the inferior vena cava (the vein that transports blood from your lower body to your heart). Back-sleeping can also put you at risk of backache, piles, indigestion, breathing difficulties and circulation and blood-pressure changes. Instead, lie on your side, preferably your left side. Although there's no harm in sleeping on your right side, lying on your left side is beneficial for you and your baby: it improves the flow of blood and nutrients to the placenta and helps your kidneys eliminate waste products and excess fluid. That, in turn, reduces swelling in your ankles, feet and hands. If you wake up and find yourself on your stomach or back, don't worry.

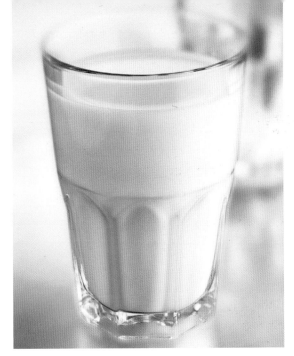

BEDTIME DRINK *The amino acid l-tryptophan (found in milk and other foods, such as turkey and eggs) is thought to make the eyelids heavy by raising the level of a chemical in the brain called serotonin.*

I'm tense and overtired and can't sleep once I get to bed. What can I do to relax?

You need to calm your mind and relax your muscles to sleep soundly. Try some gentle yoga (see pp 146–7) and stretching exercises – but nothing too vigorous, as exercising before bedtime can keep you awake. Breathing deeply and rhythmically can ease muscle tension, lower your heart rate and help you to fall asleep.

Finally, try guided imagery. Picture yourself in a quiet, relaxing scene, such as a warm sandy beach. Imagine every detail, including the sounds, smells, tastes, and textures. It may take some practice, but guided imagery can calm your restless or anxious mind and aid sleep.

Is it safe to use complementary therapies to help me sleep?

Certain essential oils, such as lavender, can help you to get a good night's sleep, especially when combined with a base oil for a relaxing massage before bed. However, essential oils should only be used during pregnancy under the supervision of a registered aromatherapist. Herbal remedies come in many forms, including fresh or dried plants, pills, tinctures, and powders. Although herbs are considered natural alternatives to certain drugs, they can be equally powerful or even toxic. Talk to a registered herbalist before taking any herbal remedy in pregnancy.

I've been having strange dreams. Is this normal during pregnancy?

Yes, if your dreams seem more bizarre than usual, filled with images of sex, talking animals, and huge, towering buildings, you can put them down to a combination of progesterone surging through your veins and your excitement and apprehension about pregnancy and motherhood. Another reason why your dreams may have changed is that you are more likely to interrupt a dream-filled cycle of REM sleep by frequent waking during the night.

JUST FOR DAD

What dads-to-be dream about
Your feelings of excitement, anticipation and anxiety may open a floodgate of dreams.

***First trimester:** You may have more sexual dreams. This could be because the protective feelings a man develops towards his wife and unborn child may be threatening to his masculinity. Sexual dreams and other macho visions (such as footballing triumphs) may be expressing a need to be more 'masculine'.*

***Second trimester:** You may dream about your family background, or that you are pregnant and giving birth. This may be because you want to share in the pregnancy experience. Dads-to-be often feel left out at this stage of the pregnancy and may dream they are excluded and alone.*

***Third trimester:** You may dream of finding babies or of being given them, sometimes during elaborate ceremonies or rites. You may have dreams of celebrating the baby's birth. Dreams of this kind indicate acceptance and valuing of the baby.*

What causes skin and hair changes during pregnancy?

Overall, the skin and hair changes during pregnancy are positive, but you may experience some minor skin problems. Be reassured that the majority of these will disappear in the weeks following the birth of your baby.

Will I begin to 'glow' this trimester?

Yes, the 'bloom' or 'glow' of pregnancy is not just a saying. Your skin retains more moisture during pregnancy, which plumps it up, smoothing out any fine lines and wrinkles that you may have. The pinkish glow that makes you look radiant is due to increased levels of blood circulating round your body. It may also make you feel slightly flushed.

Why do I have brown patches of skin?

This is chloasma, also known as the 'mask of pregnancy', which has the appearance of brown patches of pigmentation on the forehead, cheeks and neck. On darker-skinned women, they may appear as lighter patches. It's caused by the increased production of melanin, the tanning hormone that protects the skin against ultraviolet light. Exposure to sunlight will darken the patches so protect your skin with a high factor sunscreen.

What is the dark line on my tummy?

This is called linea nigra. It is a dark, vertical line that appears down the middle of a woman's stomach during pregnancy, often crossing the navel. It tends to appear around the second trimester and is caused by pigmentation changes in the skin. There's no known reason for why the linea nigra appears where it does.

What's causing the tiny veins on my face?

These tiny clusters of broken capillaries (small blood vessels), or spider naevi as they are sometimes known, most often appear on the cheeks, and are common in pregnancy, particularly if you are already prone to them. They are caused by the increased volume of circulating blood putting extra pressure on the capillaries, which are also more sensitive during pregnancy. To reduce the chances of spider naevi appearing, protect your face from extremes of cold or heat, as exposure to either can encourage the problem.

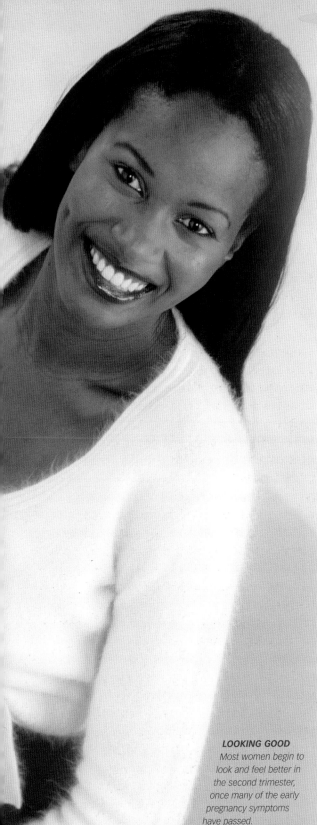

LOOKING GOOD
Most women begin to look and feel better in the second trimester, once many of the early pregnancy symptoms have passed.

Why am I breaking out in spots?

Pregnancy can sometimes trigger acne. Higher levels of hormones encourage the production of sebum – the oil that keeps our skin supple – but this can cause the pores to become blocked. Don't use acne creams without seeking medical advice.

Can I prevent stretch marks?

You can't prevent stretch marks, but you can try to minimize them. Rub oil or cream rich in vitamin E on your bump to keep the skin supple. Avoid putting weight on too quickly by eating a healthy diet (see pp 48–9) and doing gentle exercise (see pp 56–7).

Should I be worried about itchy skin?

Some itchiness is quite common, but in the third trimester itchy skin can be a sign of a serious liver problem called obstetric cholestasis. Seek medical advice if your itchiness is severe and particularly if it affects the soles of your feet and your palms.

My hair is wonderfully thick. Why is this?

You're not growing more hair; you're just losing less than normal due to pregnancy hormones. If you normally have a thick head of hair and worry that any more will be unmanageable, you may find a shorter cut easier to deal with. But don't do anything that you may regret; you're going through enough change as it is.

QUICK TIP

Taking a folic acid supplement and eating foods rich in folates, such as whole grains, chicken and beef liver, and leafy green vegetables can reduce pigmentation changes such as chloasma and linea nigra (see left).

Should my diet change now that I'm in the second trimester?

Like most pregnant women, you'll probably find that your morning sickness passes and your appetite returns around the beginning of the second trimester. Your diet should include key foods that fuel your baby's development and keep you healthy.

Do I need to worry about the fat content of my diet?

Yes, you should monitor your fat intake to ensure that no more than 30 per cent of your daily calories come from fat. But don't feel guilty if you indulge in a bag of crisps or a portion of chips occasionally – you can make up for it by trying to stick to lower-fat foods the following day. You should try to get about four servings of fat a day. Ideally these should be monounsaturated fats, found in olive, rapeseed and peanut oils, as well as in nuts and nut butters, or polyunsaturated fats – these include the omega-3 fatty acids found in some oily fish, such as sardines, mackerel and herring.

The worst fats are saturated fats found in high-fat meats and whole milk (skimmed and semi-skimmed milk will provide sufficient calcium), and hydrogenated fats found in margarine, biscuits, crisps and many ready-made foods.

What's the best way to get a good intake of iron and how much should I have?

All women (whether pregnant or not) should aim to have over 14 mg of iron per day. Lean red meat is the richest source – the iron in animal sources is absorbed easily by the body. There is also iron in pulses, dried fruit, green leafy vegetables, nuts and seeds, and in fortified breakfast cereals and breads, but the iron in these foods is not so easily absorbed.

To pump up your iron intake, cut back on coffee and tea because natural substances in these drinks reduce the amount of iron your body absorbs. If nothing else, make sure you don't have these drinks at mealtimes or until half an hour after eating iron-rich foods or taking an iron supplement. Steam vegetables, or use only a small amount of water, to prevent iron being lost during cooking (as well as the vitamin C that is needed to absorb iron). Calcium decreases iron absorption, so don't take your supplement with a glass of milk or while you're eating dairy products and other high-calcium foods.

ASK THE EXPERT
FIONA FORD
DIETICIAN

I've been diagnosed with gestational diabetes. How should I adapt my diet?

If you have gestational diabetes, one way to keep your blood sugar levels under control is to follow a specific meal plan. A dietician will work out how many calories you need each day. Then she'll teach you how to measure portion sizes and how to balance your meals with just the right amounts of protein, carbohydrates and fat. She'll also scrutinize your current diet. The five key things to remember are to eat a variety of foods, don't skip meals, eat a good breakfast, eat plenty of high-fibre foods and limit your intake of sugary foods and drinks. If dietary changes aren't enough to keep your blood sugar in a healthy range, you'll need to take insulin under medical guidance.

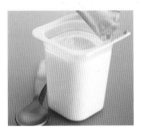
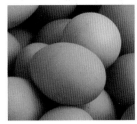
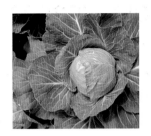
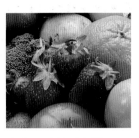

GOOD FOR YOU AND YOUR BABY *Dairy products and well-cooked eggs are great sources of protein and green leafy vegetables provide essential iron. If you're hungry between meals, try to snack on a healthy piece of fruit rather than reach for a biscuit or packet of crisps.*

Should I be eating lots of dairy products?

It depends on how much you normally consume. While you can get the same nutrients from other food groups, dairy products are excellent sources of calcium, protein, vitamin D and phosphorous – nutrients important for your baby's developing bones and teeth, muscles, heart and nerves, and for blood-clotting. Aim to eat three to four servings of calcium-rich foods a day during pregnancy, enough to give you 1,000 mg. Choose low- or non-fat dairy products whenever possible – you'll get all the nutrients without the added fat. It may be beneficial for women who don't eat dairy foods to take a calcium supplement.

Is it safe to take omega-3 fish oil supplements during pregnancy?

Yes and no. There are two types of fish oil supplement – those that are made from the liver of the fish and those that are made from the body of the fish. Supplements made from the liver, such as cod liver oil, contain the retinol form of vitamin A and need to be either avoided altogether or strictly limited during pregnancy so that your daily intake does not exceed 3,300 micrograms (mcg). On the other hand, fish oils that are not derived from fish livers contain lots of omega-3 fatty acids. These are essential for your baby's developing eyes and brain, but do choose a supplement suitable for pregnancy.

Why is it so important to drink water?

None of your organs could function without water and your body uses even more water during pregnancy. Among other things, it's needed to make the plasma essential for your expanding blood volume and to form the amniotic fluid that bathes and cushions your developing baby.

You also need water to help flush out waste, which in turn can help to prevent bladder infections. If you drink plenty of water, your urine will stay diluted and you'll urinate more often – thus lessening the chance that bacteria will hang around in your bladder and multiply. What's more, drinking plenty of water can help to ward off constipation and help to prevent piles (see pp 144–5), which are both common complaints during pregnancy.

Believe it or not, the more water you drink while you are pregnant, the less water your body will retain and the less likely you are to be plagued by swollen hands and feet (see pp 92–3) as your pregnancy progresses.

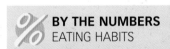

BY THE NUMBERS
EATING HABITS

How many times a day do you eat?

30% *5 times a day.*

26% *4 times a day.*

23% *6 times a day or more.*

16% *3 times a day.*

5% *2 times a day.*

Source: A BabyCenter.com poll of more than 32,000 pregnant women.

Why am I having food cravings?

The majority of pregnant women experience a craving for certain foods at some point in their pregnancy. While it's okay to indulge in unhealthy foods occasionally, if this is all you want to eat, it's important to find a way to control your cravings so that your overall diet remains nutritious and balanced.

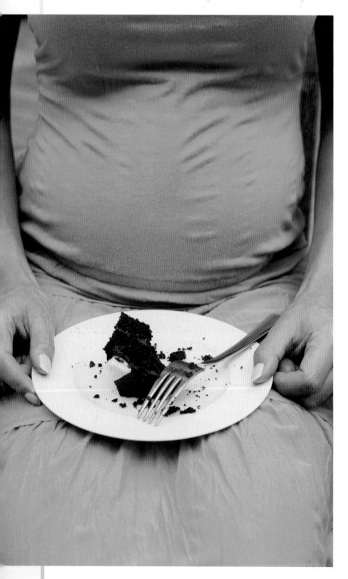

I've had cravings for particular foods since being pregnant. Is this normal?

Yes, what you're experiencing is very common during pregnancy. Yearning for a particular type of food is an undeniable part of carrying a baby. In fact, about 85 per cent of expectant mothers report at least one major food craving. These cravings often seem to come out of nowhere and have an overpowering ferocity. Some of the most commonly craved foods are chocolate, citrus fruits, pickles, chips and ice cream. The most common aversions are to coffee, tea, fried or fatty foods, highly spiced foods, meat and eggs. Experts are still mystified about exactly what causes the phenomenon – no one knows for sure whether cravings are related to hormonal changes or emotional issues or some combination of these. It does seem that hormonal changes can have a powerful impact on taste and smell, but experts are sceptical that food cravings can be attributed simply to hormones.

Is craving a food a sign that your diet is deficient in a certain area?

Some alternative medicine practitioners believe that a craving for chocolate may be triggered by a shortage of B vitamins. Similarly, a craving for red meat seems like a transparent cry for protein. Still, the link between what your body needs and what you crave seems weak. If it were strong we would all be craving broccoli and fresh fruit, rather than the chocolate and crisps most of us seem to be desperate to eat.

Should I try to be stronger and not give in to my food cravings?

It really depends what you're craving. While a few pregnant women have been known to pine for broccoli, spinach or bananas, most reach for ice cream and chocolate. If your urge for sugar and fat is just too powerful to resist, go ahead and indulge occasionally. But think, too, of the nutrients your growing baby needs (see pp 52–3) and try to work them into your sugar or salt fix.

Can you suggest any ways to control my unhealthy food cravings?

Yes, there are a few ways you can keep the urges at bay. Eat breakfast every day, as this will make you less susceptible to mid-morning junk-food snack attacks. Exercise regularly – working out is an excellent way to curb cravings for unhealthy foods (and the boredom or anxiety that can lead to excessive snacking). Get the emotional support you need. The hormonal roller coaster of pregnancy can make you more vulnerable to mood swings and you may turn to food when what you really need is someone to talk to. Train yourself to think small. Try a few spoonfuls of ice cream rather than a whole bowl, or one square of chocolate instead of the entire bar. Or if you find those mini portions are just too much of a tease, have a normal portion, but try to do so less often.

What causes the cravings for non-food items and is it harmful?

No one knows for sure what causes this common phenomenon. It is called pica after the Latin for magpie, a bird that will eat almost anything. The range of items craved really is bizarre: examples include dirt, ashes, clay, chalk, ice, baking soda, soap, toothpaste, paint chips, plaster, wax, hair and even cigarette butts. In some studies, these cravings have been linked to an iron deficiency – even though none of the craved items contains significant amounts of iron. But if you crave any of these items, that doesn't necessarily mean you have any sort of deficiency, and it definitely doesn't mean you should eat them! In fact, eating non-food substances can interfere with nutrient absorption and may cause a deficiency. And while eating ice is not likely to be harmful, eating dirt or most of the other items mentioned can lead to illness. If you are having any strong cravings for non-food items, talk to your midwife. It's worth getting checked for any underlying physical or psychological problem.

IF YOU DO NOTHING ELSE...

- *Monitor what you're eating and aim for only small amounts of any unhealthy foods you crave.*
- *Stay busy to reduce the boredom that can often lead to temptation.*
- *Seek medical advice if you crave non-food items.*

Am I putting on the right amount of weight?

The range of pregnancy weight gain that's considered normal is fairly wide, so don't become too focused on the extra pounds you're gaining, and remember your weight will be monitored by your midwife at antenatal checks. In general, you just need to avoid extremes of gaining too much or too little weight.

I'm worried I'm gaining too much weight. What's normal?

Every woman is individual so it isn't possible to estimate what you will gain. The average weight gain is about 11 kg (24.2 lb), but the amount you gain will depend on how heavy you were before you became pregnant or more accurately, on what your body mass index – BMI – was (see pp 54–5). It is important to accept that you are going to put on weight. You are meant to because your body is changing to give your baby the best start in life. Remember, most of the weight comes from your baby and his support system (see box, right).

ASK THE EXPERT
FIONA FORD
DIETICIAN

Is it true there's a link between pregnancy weight gain and breast cancer?

Not directly, but research shows that women who put on a lot of weight during pregnancy and don't lose it afterwards are more likely to become obese. In later life, this will make them more susceptible to obesity-related diseases, such as diabetes, heart disease and cancer, including breast cancer. Experts recommend that women should pay attention to their lifestyle during pregnancy and especially to taking regular exercise (see pp 56–7). It's also a good idea to try to lose any excess 'baby weight' after having your baby (see pp 212–3).

Should I be eating for two?

Your body becomes more efficient when you're expecting a baby and makes even better use of the energy you obtain from food. The average woman does not need any extra calories for the first six months of pregnancy and only about 200 extra calories per day for the last three months. This number of calories is equivalent to: two slices of wholemeal toast with margarine or butter; a jacket potato with 28 g (1 oz) of cheese; or one slice of cheese on toast.

I've always had weight issues. How will I cope with the extra amount I'm gaining?

If you've struggled with your weight or body image in the past, you may have a hard time accepting that it's okay to gain weight now. It's normal to feel anxious as the numbers on the scales creep up, but the weight you gain during pregnancy is vital to your baby's health. In fact, not gaining enough weight increases the odds that your baby also won't gain weight properly and could be born prematurely.

I'm a diabetic. Do I need to be particularly careful about what I eat?

Yes, it's especially important that you start pregnancy with a healthy BMI (see pp 54–5). Babies born to diabetic mothers can grow very large and

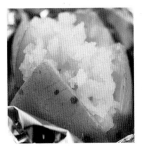 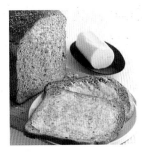

EXTRA CALORIES *In the final months of pregnancy, try to eat an extra 200 calories per day. Good sources are a jacket potato with cheese, or a couple of slices of bread and butter.*

there is a risk to the baby's health if blood sugar levels are not kept at a stable level. You should ask your carers for advice on the best possible diet to keep yourself and your baby healthy. Most maternity hospitals have a special team of doctors and nurses who are specially trained to look after diabetic women in pregnancy.

How quickly will I lose the weight once the baby is born?

While you probably won't return to your pre-pregnancy size for some time, you will lose a significant amount of weight immediately after the birth, when you've lost the weight of your baby and his support system (see right).

The weight keeps coming off, too. Throughout pregnancy, your body's cells were hard at work retaining water to build up your blood volume and make amniotic fluid, and now all that extra fluid will be excreted.

You'll produce more urine than usual in the days after birth and you may perspire more than usual. By the end of the first week, you'll lose about 1.8 kg (4 lb) of water weight, depending on how much water you retained during pregnancy. How quickly you then continue to lose weight will depend on lifestyle factors, such as how much you exercise (see pp 212–3) and your diet.

JUST THE FACTS
WHERE THE WEIGHT GOES

Your baby and his support system make up most of your weight gain. Here's an approximate guide:

- *At birth, your baby will weigh approximately 3.3 kg (7.3 lb).*
- *During pregnancy, the muscle layer of your uterus grows dramatically and weighs an extra 900 g (2 lb).*
- *The placenta, which keeps your baby nourished, weighs 600 g (1.3 lb).*
- *Your breasts weigh an extra 400 g (0.9 lb).*
- *Your blood volume increases and weighs an extra 1.2 kg (2.6 lb).*
- *You have extra fluid in your body, weighing 2.6 kg (5.7 lb).*
- *You lay down about 2.5 kg (5.5 lb) extra fat to provide you with extra energy for breastfeeding.*

BabyCentre Buzz

"I'm a little alarmed at how big and bumbling I already feel. I've never gained so much weight so quickly, and I hate how big my bum and thighs are getting. Two things keep me from getting too depressed, though: knowing that this weight gain is normal and good for my baby, and that my husband loves my extra padding!" Georgie

"I'm trying very hard to surrender to the reality of the weight I'm gaining now that I'm pregnant, and trust that my body will allow me to lose the weight after I have the baby. I certainly feel much better since throwing out my scales!" Deanna

"My midwife has told me not to worry too much about weight gain. She assured me that if she thought I was putting on too much weight, then she would tell me and advise me appropriately." Natalene

Is it still safe to exercise?

As long as you don't have health complications it's safe to exercise throughout pregnancy, and the second trimester is often the best time to take on a regular routine. And, remember, the time you invest now in improving or maintaining your fitness is likely to pay off when you are in the delivery room in a few months' time.

Will I need to change my exercise routine now that I'm in the second trimester?

Yes. Even if you were active before your pregnancy, you will naturally feel inclined to scale down your exercise routine to accommodate your growing uterus. During the first trimester it's especially important that you avoid overheating (see p 57). After the first trimester, you'll also need to eliminate exercises that are performed while flat on your back or while you're standing in one place for long periods, as both can reduce blood flow to the baby.

ASK THE EXPERT
ALISON BOURNE
PHYSIOTHERAPIST

Is it safe to continue weight-training exercises now that I'm pregnant?

Yes, but you'll need to avoid certain positions, such as forcefully pushing or exerting pressure while holding your breath; this can affect blood pressure. You'll need to work with weights no heavier than 2.2 kg (5 lb), but you can do more repetitions. One set of 12 for each muscle group is safe. It's a good idea to go over your regime with your doctor, midwife or a physiotherapist first. In the second trimester, avoid lifting weights while standing. Because you have an increase in blood volume, blood vessel walls are more stretchy, which can cause variations in blood flow and leave you feeling lightheaded. Always tighten your pelvic floor (see right) before lifting weights.

How can I tell if I'm exercising too much?

In general, you shouldn't go for the burn or exercise to exhaustion. Because you'll have less oxygen available for aerobic exercise and because your heart is working harder than normal, you should generally stick to 60 per cent of your maximum heart rate while pregnant. Some women like to monitor their heart rate while exercising, but you should never rely on this alone as heart rates in pregnancy can vary widely. It is safer to be guided by how you are feeling. A good rule of thumb is to slow down if you can't comfortably carry on a conversation while exercising. And stop exercising immediately if you experience any of the following: dizziness, shortness of breath, chest pain, feeling faint, vaginal bleeding or leaking of amniotic fluid, difficulty walking, contractions or unusual absence of fetal movements. But do bear in mind that your baby is often most quiet when you're exercising.

Why is walking good during pregnancy?

Walking keeps you fit without jarring your knees and ankles. It's also a safe activity throughout the nine months of pregnancy and one of the easier ways to start exercising if you are not a regular exerciser. If you've been walking, keep it up. If you were fairly inactive before you became pregnant, start with a slow walk and build yourself up to brisk 20- to 30-minute jaunts. You could alternate a few minutes at a brisk pace with a few minutes at a slower pace. As you get bigger, you may start to feel more ungainly, and may even begin to waddle. Pay attention to your posture when you walk and swing your arms for balance, to stabilize your pelvis and to intensify your workout.

Can I still go to my aerobics class?

Yes, as long as you choose exercises that are low impact. This mean no high kicks and leaps to minimize stress on the joints and your pelvic floor. You should be able to continue your routine throughout your pregnancy, gradually tapering off towards the end. Although you could also stay fit at home with the help of an exercise video, it's best if you choose a class especially designed for expectant mothers.

What are pelvic floor exercises?

The pelvic floor muscles help to hold the bladder, uterus and bowel in place and to control the muscles that close the anus, vagina and urethra. When the pelvic floor muscles are weakened it can result in stress incontinence, which means you leak small amounts of urine while coughing, sneezing, laughing or exercising. This is common in late pregnancy and after childbirth. Pelvic floor exercises can strengthen these muscles. Strong pelvic floor muscles support the extra weight of pregnancy and help in the second stage of labour. To do a pelvic floor exercise, imagine that you are trying to stop yourself from passing wind and trying to stop your flow of urine, at the same time. Hold for up to 10 seconds without holding your breath, then release and rest for a few seconds. Repeat up to 10 times.

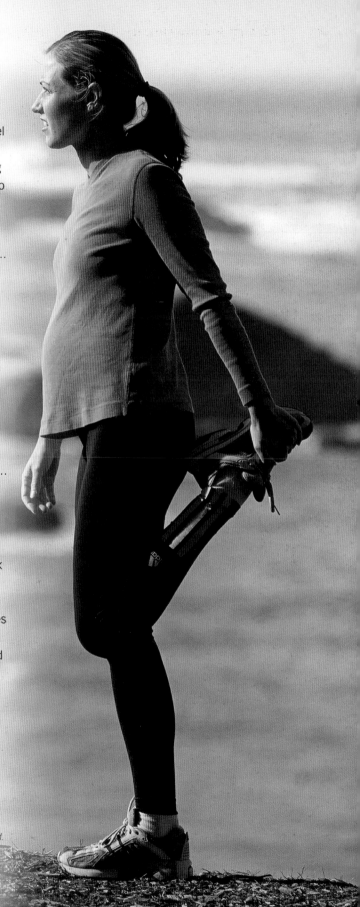

STAIRS FIT *There is no reason why you can't continue to enjoy a favourite pastime, such as jogging, just because you're pregnant. However, take it easy – now is not the time to push yourself too hard.*

How can we decide on a name for our baby?

Deciding on a name for your baby can be fun, but also incredibly frustrating! It's best to start thinking about it around halfway through your pregnancy and try lots of different combinations. Don't be surprised if you and your partner change your minds often; just make sure you're settled on something by the time your baby is born.

My partner and I just can't seem to agree on a name. What should we do?

If choosing a name is hard for one parent, hitting upon something you both like can be even trickier. It can come as a blow if you've grown up loving a particular name, and have been planning to bestow it on your firstborn, only for your partner to reject it out of hand; or if he's determined to give your son a footballing name when you can't stand sport. One way of avoiding this is to draw up a list of possibilities while you're still pregnant. Have a column for girls and another for boys. Go down the list marking your likes and dislikes and get your partner to do the same. Then draw up a shortlist. Refer to it often, as your feelings may change. If you have more than one favourite between you, you could always compromise by using one as a middle name. When you're choosing names, also be aware of undesirable initial combinations such as SAD.

No one seems to like the name we've chosen. Should we change it?

Once you've settled on a name that you both like, it can be disheartening when other people are less than enthusiastic. Insensitive individuals might even say outright that they don't like your choice. But it's an entirely personal decision and you will never be able to please everyone, so don't change your mind because of other people. It's harder if a family member isn't keen, as you might imagine them cringing each time they have to call your child by their name, but whether you change your mind is down to you. Remember that names grow on people, and once your child is known by his or her name, everyone will get used to it. The alternative is not to tell anyone the name you have chosen – many parents-to-be do this – so that you don't have to deal with the reactions of other people.

The boy's name we like is already very popular. Should we rethink?

Names do go in and out of fashion, and the problem with choosing a popular name is that your child may be one of many in his social circle. If, for instance,

---

JUST THE FACTS
REGISTERING THE BIRTH

- *Your baby's birth must be registered within six weeks in England, Northern Ireland and Wales and within three weeks in Scotland.*

- *Make sure you're certain about your baby's name because if you change it – even the spelling – a new certificate has to be issued.*

- *If you are married, only one of you needs to register the birth, but if you are not married and the father wants his name on the certificate you both have to attend.*

you name him Jack, you may find that he's one of many Jacks in his class. He may then end up being known by his whole name, or having his surname initial tacked on to the end of his first name.

We're being pressured to give our son a family name. What should we do?

'Family names' can be archaic and odd-sounding because of the length of the tradition, or perhaps just not to your taste. In some cultures, it's expected that a child will be named after his parents, grandparents or other relative, whether the name is a favourite of yours or not. Both situations can be tricky, but there are ways of breaking with tradition without giving offence. You could 'bury' the name by using it as a middle name. If you do use it as your child's first name, you could devise a more modern-sounding spelling or nickname from it.

We're from different cultures. How can we find the right name for our baby?

If you and your partner come from different cultural backgrounds, it's worth trying to merge the two as it can help to give children a sense of both sides of their roots. If, for instance, your husband is Greek and you are English, you may be able to compromise by choosing a Greek name that is easily pronounceable in English, such as Anna for a girl. Or you could choose a name that has an English equivalent (eg. George for Georgios). You could also choose a first name from one culture and a middle name from the other. Experiment with different combinations until you find one that works.

Do middle names really matter?

Middle names are optional, but they do help to single your child out from others who have the same first and last names. This could be the place

BabyCentre Buzz

"Remember to consider the spelling of a name as well. My mum spelled my name 'Sahra'. This is pronounced Sara NOT Sarah. All my life I've had people ask if I've spelled it correctly. Please think about unusual spellings, all mums- and dads-to-be. It just makes the kid's life a little bit easier." Sahra

"I have this thing about people looking like their names, so I am afraid that my first two children were nameless for three days! Some people think that I am a bit mad for feeling this way, but it has worked out well for us. The two of them seem to fit their names very well personality-wise." Miki

"I had my kids in the 1980s and I named them – wait for it – Kylie and Jayson. I really regret it and I have advice for other parents: definitely don't decide to name your child after 'in' people!" Monique

for a beloved grandparent's name or even one from each side of the family. You may be able to trace some of your family tree and find an ancestor with an unusual, attractive name, to give your child a sense of history; or you may want to honour your best friend, favourite teacher, sporting hero or even midwife! Some children grow up disliking their first names, and opt to use their middle names, instead, so it's worth bearing this in mind.

I'm expecting twins. How can I find suitable names?

When it comes to naming twins, there are no hard and fast rules. Some people choose names which begin with the same letter, others choose names which have the same number of syllables. You could consider using themes. For example, Lily and Poppy are both names of flowers; Elijah and Joel are both names meaning 'God' in Hebrew.

My clothes are beginning to feel very tight. What am I going to wear?

You don't necessarily have to spend lots of money on maternity clothes. There are many ways to adapt the clothes you have and mix and match items so that you stay looking good and feeling comfortable throughout your pregnancy.

I can't afford to buy many maternity clothes. What essential items do I need?

No woman wants to wear the same thing over and over again, especially if she's feeling fed up and fatter than usual. And as you're pregnant for nine months – that's at least two different seasons of weather as well as two different seasons of fashion. Nevertheless, you can get away with investing in just a few 'key' items of maternity wear that can be mixed and matched. Try two pairs of well-cut trousers, a plain skirt or dress, a cardigan or jacket, a plain jumper that can be worn over most outfits, two casual tops and a smart top. What you buy also depends on how you feel about showing your bump. Some women prefer to cover up, while others are proud to show it off.

How can I adapt the clothes I already have to fit my new shape?

Before your bump becomes too big, you can make do with your existing clothes by wearing longer tops – hiding the fact that you've left the top button undone on your trousers. Later on in pregnancy, with a bit of crafty needlework, you could use buttons and fabric panels or strips to temporarily expand your favourite clothes. Again, those longer tops will come in handy. When elasticated waists feel like they're groaning under the strain of your tummy, you could replace them with a drawstring.

I love jeans but can't find any to fit me now that I'm pregnant. Any tips?

Try men's jeans. If you can find the right size, they'll sit nicely under your bump, avoiding that unattractive high-waisted look and eliminating the need for frumpy elasticated panels. And don't stop there when it comes to raiding your partner's wardrobe! If you're just slouching around the house,

BabyCentre Buzz

"My friend who had her baby before me gave me all her unwanted maternity clothes. I'm not really a fan of second-hand stuff or 'hand-me-downs', but it was really nice of her, and useful." Sharon

"You should try looking on eBay if you don't want to shell out loads of money for new clothes. They always have lots of maternity stuff for sale!" Jodi

"My advice is to wear your bump with pride! After spending years trying to hold in my stomach, I was finally proud to be sticking it out!" Sarah

"I missed my bump like I never thought possible after I'd given birth to my daughter, so all you soon-to-be mums stick it out and be proud of your baby. I can't wait to do it all again." Elizabeth

wear his shirts and jumpers – and the elasticated waist on men's boxer shorts and pyjama bottoms makes them comfortable to wear in bed.

How can I dress well for work?

For the first trimester, you'll probably be able to wear your usual clothes. You may have to leave the top button undone, but you can hide that by leaving your shirts untucked. When your waistband gets tight, loop a rubber band through the buttonhole and then wrap it around the button for extra breathing space. If you find your breasts grow quickly, opt for loose tops or wear suit jackets open over a T-shirt or shirt. Once you're a bit big for your normal clothes, buy trousers and skirts with elasticated or drawstring waistbands in a size larger than you usually wear.

Is it true that I can't wear high heels?

High heels alter your posture and put a strain on your lower back. The ligaments that control this area are softened in pregnancy so it's more likely that they can be stretched and damaged. Add to that the additional weight of your growing baby and the combination of baby and high heels could contribute to lower back pain, which can be severe. Flatter shoes are a better bet on a day-to-day basis. Keep your high heels for high days and holidays, and slip a pair of flatties in your bag so you can change into something more comfortable.

My most comfortable clothes are really bland. What can I do?

Simply accessorize! Beads, bangles, bags, ribbons, scarves, shoes ... the possibilities are endless. You can dress an outfit up or down to suit both occasion and mood, and you can still wear your new accessories after your baby is born.

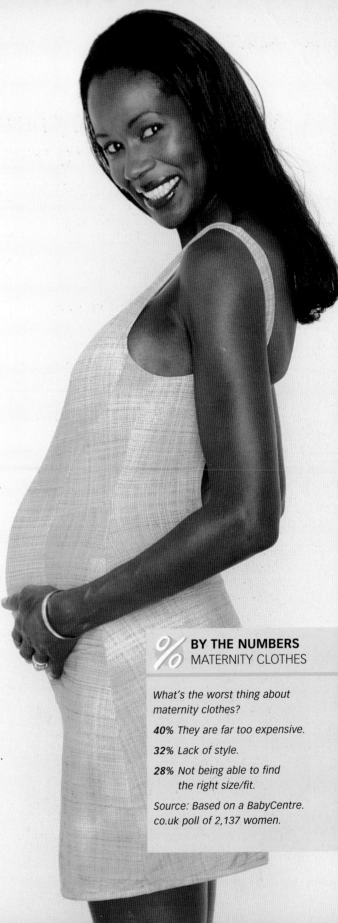

% BY THE NUMBERS
MATERNITY CLOTHES

What's the worst thing about maternity clothes?

40% *They are far too expensive.*

32% *Lack of style.*

28% *Not being able to find the right size/fit.*

Source: Based on a BabyCentre. co.uk poll of 2,137 women.

How can we keep our relationship on track?

Once you're safely into the second trimester, your pregnancy will become much more real to you and your partner. You are bound to feel excited and want to make plans for your baby's arrival. However, it's also important to make sure the pregnancy doesn't take over to the detriment of your relationship.

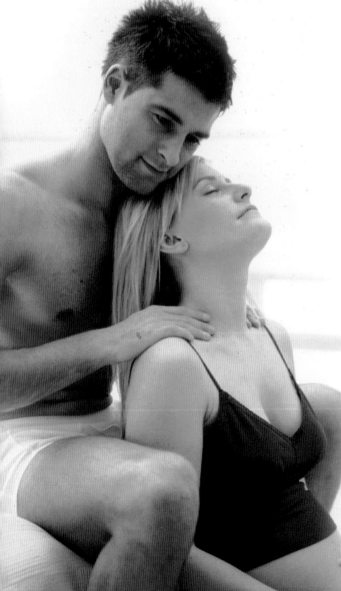

I feel like we only ever talk about the pregnancy now. How can we maintain our identity as a couple?

It's normal for the pregnancy to take over, especially if it's your first baby. The key is to ensure that you make time to share interests other than your pregnancy, too. You're still a couple, after all, not just parents-to-be – and it's this closeness that will keep your relationship and your family healthy in the years ahead. When you go out, for example, agree to talk about the pregnancy for only a set amount of time. Make a game of it, with the person who returns to the subject receiving a forfeit!

I've felt quite alone up to now. Why has it taken my partner so long to come to terms with the pregnancy?

The reality of your pregnancy has probably taken some time to sink in because it's not physically happening to your partner. Besides, up to now you've looked the same on the outside. Many men start becoming more involved and excited once the bump is there as visible proof. It's normal for it to finally hit home when that happens. Your partner will probably become completely fascinated by your changing shape. Treat your partner's new awareness as an opportunity to get closer and plan together for the big event.

BabyCentre Buzz

"At 20 weeks, I was at my wit's end. My husband had no idea how to relate to me. But now he's made an about-turn. I think it just took him a little while to get used to the fact that I was pregnant, then suddenly it became 'real' to him." Jessica

"My husband was great before we got pregnant, but now he's just unbelievable. He's forever cleaning the house, cooking dinner, running errands – and has never once complained. I don't know what I'd do without him." Lisa

"At first my husband didn't seem to want anything to do with my pregnancy, so I made sure he came along to all my antenatal appointments and ultrasounds. It made a big difference once he saw our son's image on the monitor." Amber

The months are passing so quickly. How can we make the most of our time as a couple before we become 'three'?

Becoming parents needn't and shouldn't spell the end of time together for just the two of you – but there is no denying that it will take some organizing. So enjoy the chance of 'alone' time now, while the going is good. Forget your roles as parents-to-be for a few hours, and just enjoy being a couple. It's easy to get so caught up in work, baby preparations, and other responsibilities that you forget to make time for each other. Make a point of setting aside a regular time each week for just that.

Now is also the perfect time to take a holiday (see pp 120–1). You're feeling better, your due date is still several months away, and you don't have too many antenatal appointments keeping you close to home. It may also be some time before you go away again once your baby is born.

JUST FOR DAD

How to 'be there' for your partner

Be enthusiastic: Show your interest in the momentous changes going on and talk to your baby – he or she really can hear you! Try to make it to at least some of your partner's antenatal appointments, especially for the important tests, and don't be shy about asking questions. And, of course, attend antenatal classes (see pp 132–3) if you can.

Get healthier: As your partner tries to eat well and kick bad habits, support her by sharing these changes. Avoid junk food and cut down on or eliminate alcohol. Don't smoke – not just to help her abstain but because second-hand smoke can harm your baby. Spend time walking or exercising together.

Go the extra mile: Your partner may have become intensely demanding. Accept it. She's doing all the hard work, so do the supermarket run, acquaint yourself with the vacuum, send her flowers, and do your best to indulge her midnight demands for cottage cheese and jam – with a smile.

Love your partner's changing body: As her pregnancy progresses, your partner may feel unattractive at times, so keep reassuring her that she's beautiful. Don't hold back on your affection. She needs hugs and kisses now more than ever.

Get busy: By the time your baby arrives, you and your partner will have bought baby clothes, prepared the nursery, bought and installed a car seat ... and you thought you had nothing to do!

I'm more inclined to share my pregnancy with my sister than partner. Why is this?

Many women feel that their partner just doesn't 'get it' when it comes to pregnancy, which is why they talk more to their female relatives and friends. A man's perspective is understandably different. Nobody who's not pregnant can fully comprehend the minute-by-minute, close-to-the-heart reality of carrying a baby inside your body. But that doesn't mean your partner has to be a bystander; there are plenty of ways he can participate (see above).

I've rediscovered my libido. Is this normal?

It's normal to feel in the mood for lovemaking again once the early pregnancy symptoms have passed and, if you don't have any pregnancy complications, you can enjoy a healthy sex life. As your pregnancy progresses, you may begin to dislike your body, but be reassured that many men find their partners just as attractive.

I'm feeling so much better now and can't get enough sex. Is there something wrong with me?

No, the return of your libido is completely normal. After the exhaustion and nausea of the first trimester finally pass, it's not uncommon to feel your sexual desire skyrocket. You can thank the increased bloodflow to your pelvic area and the heightened sensitivity to stimulation this brings about, as well as those ever-active hormones that contribute to increased vaginal lubrication. If your partner's passion matches your revved-up libido, just go for it!

BabyCentre Buzz

"When I first got pregnant I was too scared to have sex, but now that I'm in week 14 I'm relieved to say I'm more relaxed and enjoying it again." Tara

"Wow, I love sex in pregnancy! I can't get enough of it – my sex drive is definitely higher than it has ever been. My poor partner is more tired than me, though of course he isn't complaining!" Julie

"My husband doesn't want sex at all, even though I am a very nice-looking pregnant woman! I think he is scared of harming the baby, even though I've told him there is no risk." Rebecca

Now that I'm in the mood for having sex, my partner seems to have gone off it. Why is this?

Try not to be crushed if you find your partner's lust waning just when you're raring to go again. As your belly blossoms, his fear of hurting you or your baby becomes more real. Unless your midwife has told you otherwise, reassure him that lovemaking is perfectly safe and that you'll speak up if anything feels uncomfortable. If that doesn't allay his concerns, take him along to your next antenatal appointment so your midwife can put his mind at ease. Another worry for some men is the notion that a mother isn't an appropriate sexual partner. Talk openly about his feelings without pressuring him. Let him know that you still need to see each other as lovers even though you're also going to become parents.

My partner and I have always enjoyed using sex toys. Can we continue to do this now that I'm pregnant?

Unfortunately, there's been no research in this area, but if using sex toys is a normal part of your sex life, there should be no reason for you to stop using them if you have a healthy, uncomplicated pregnancy. Just take care to keep any sex toys clean and don't mix orifices. Do not penetrate too forcefully, since plastic is more rigid than flesh.

JUST THE FACTS
SEX POSITIONS DURING PREGNANCY

Where there's a will, there's a way! With a little experimenting, you and your partner will find a sexual position that works for you. Try the following variations:

- *Lie sideways. Lying partly sideways allows your partner to keep most of his weight off your uterus.*

- *Use the bed as a prop. Your bump isn't an obstacle if you lie on your back at the side or foot of the bed with your knees bent, and your bottom and feet perched at the edge of the mattress. Your partner can either kneel or stand in front of you.*

- *Lie side-by-side in the spoons position, which allows for only shallow penetration. Deep thrusts can become uncomfortable later in pregnancy.*

- *Get on top of your partner. It puts no weight on your abdomen and allows you to control the depth of penetration. You might also want to try sitting on your partner's lap as he sits on a sturdy chair.*

If you're diagnosed with placenta praevia (see p 37), using a sex toy (or, for that matter, having intercourse) could traumatize the placenta and cause heavy bleeding that could jeopardize your pregnancy. Other reasons to avoid sex in pregnancy include a weak cervix, abdominal cramps and bleeding.

Is it safe to give each other oral sex now that I'm pregnant?

Receiving oral sex during pregnancy is okay and if you're giving oral sex, there's no danger to the baby from the semen itself. As long as you're in a monogamous relationship and know that your partner is free of sexually transmitted diseases (STDs), there is no risk attached to having oral sex.

However, if your partner is HIV positive, it is not safe to give him oral sex because the virus will be present in his semen, and you and your developing baby could become infected (whether or not you have swallowed the semen).

I'm getting so huge and feeling really low about my body. How can my partner possibly find me attractive?

You're tired, you're sore, your stretch marks have stretch marks of their own, and it's been weeks since you could bend down to shave your legs. Do these problems sound familiar to you? If so, you're certainly not alone.

While some lucky pregnant women experience the second trimester as a time of energetic, glowing self-confidence, many others don't. However, don't worry because this feeling will pass and you will have your body back eventually. In the meantime, be kind to yourself and remember you're doing a beautiful thing – growing a baby.

Many pregnant women worry that they're no longer attractive but, believe it or not, your partner is probably loving your new shape. Be reassured that most men find their pregnant partner as attractive as ever – and often even more so (see p 67). They tend to see the sensuality in blossoming breasts and soft curves. Also, your pregnant form is a constant reminder of your partner's virility, and the new life that is growing inside you is a reminder of the bond between you.

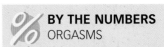

BY THE NUMBERS
ORGASMS

How did your orgasms change when you were pregnant?

48% *Felt the same as they always did.*

36% *Were more intense.*

16% *Were less intense.*

Source: A BabyCenter.com poll of more than 17,000 women.

When should I tell my employer I'm pregnant?

Most women wait until the second trimester to announce their pregnancy at work, by which time the physical changes are becoming obvious. If you intend to take maternity leave and claim Statutory Maternity Pay, there is an official week of your pregnancy by which you are legally obliged to inform your employer that you are pregnant.

When do I need to tell my employer I'm expecting a baby?

You must let your employer know about your pregnancy by the 15th week before the week that you are expecting your baby (this is called the Notification Week or the Qualification Week). Work this out by going to the Sunday before your due date (see p 21), or staying with that date if your baby is due on a Sunday, and counting back another 15 weeks.

During the notification week, you must tell your employer that you are pregnant and intend to go on maternity leave, that you want to receive Statutory Maternity Pay (SMP) (see pp 116–17) and the planned date that you will be starting your maternity leave (this cannot be earlier than 11 weeks before your due date). You can notify your employer that you are pregnant earlier if you wish but not later, or you risk losing your entitlements. Your employer will reply within 28 days, stating the date that the company expects you to return if you take your full entitlement. If you need to change the date, you will have to give 28 days' notice.

What if I receive a negative reaction to my pregnancy?

More and more employers are supportive of the work-life balance, and understand the benefits to both staff and the company. However, it is possible that you will encounter prejudices at work. Some pregnant women feel that they have to prove themselves as competent workers and end up putting in more hours than they would usually. Some find that their boss is disappointed, even angry, at their news. If this happens to you, make sure you're well-informed about your rights (see right). Stay calm, and treat the issue as you would any professional matter. Support groups, such as the Maternity Alliance (see pp 228) will be able to give you up-to-the-minute information about pregnancy and work.

Will I be entitled to maternity pay?

Depending on how long you have been in your present job, you may be entitled to Statutory Maternity Pay or Maternity Allowance (see pp 116–17). The extent of leave is also dependent on your length of service with your company. Always read your contract because you may find that you have a maternity scheme at work that gives you better rights, maternity pay and benefits than the basic package you are entitled to by law.

Can I stop working if I experience any pregnancy complications?

Talk it over with your doctor, as it will depend on your condition. You may be advised to stop if you've previously given birth to a premature baby, have

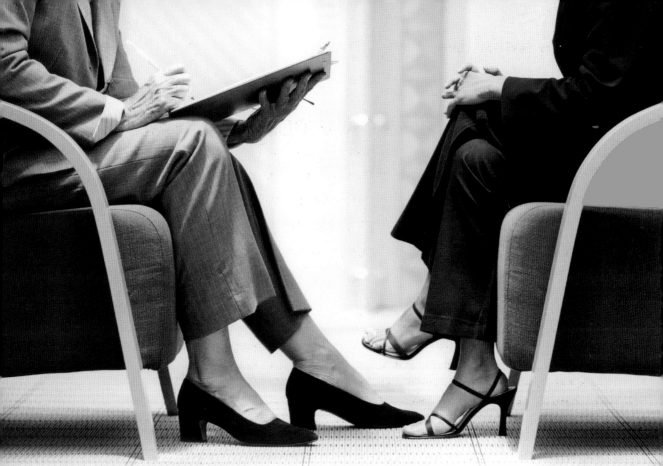

either diabetes or high blood pressure, have
a history of miscarriage or if you are expecting
more than one baby.

I'd rather have more time off once my baby is born. Can I choose to work right up to my due date?

Yes, you are allowed to choose when you want to
start your maternity leave. The only exception is if
you are sick with a pregnancy-related illness in the
last four weeks before your due date. In this case,
your employer is entitled to ask you to start your
maternity leave at once.

Towards the end of your pregnancy, you may
find yourself feeling tired very quickly, so take it as
easy as possible. And don't be a hero – if you can
afford to start your maternity leave a few weeks or
even months before your due date, consider using
it to rest, prepare and indulge yourself. Remember
that this may be the last quality time you have for
yourself for a long time to come.

JUST THE FACTS
YOUR RIGHTS

*Regardless of how long you've worked for a
company or how many hours you work, these
are your workplace rights:*

- *Your employer must carry out a workplace
  risk assessment and respect your right to
  fair treatment and time off for antenatal care.*

- *It is against the law for your employer to
  dismiss you, treat you unfairly or select you
  for redundancy for any reason connected
  with pregnancy, childbirth or maternity leave.*

- *You have the right not to be unreasonably
  refused any time off work that you need for
  antenatal care and to be paid for such time
  off. This includes time needed to travel to
  your clinic or doctor.*

*Note: Antenatal care may include parentcraft
classes, but you may need a letter from your doctor.
Your employer can ask to see an appointment card
and certificate stating that you are pregnant.*

Maternity rights: what you need to know

Make sure you are fully informed about your maternity rights so that you can maximize all the benefits that are available to you. There are legal minimums of maternity leave and pay, but always check your contract of employment as your company's policy might be more favourable.

Your entitlements

Whether you are eligible for maternity leave or pay will depend on a variety of factors, such as your length of service and your salary. Also, you may find that your company has its own maternity policy, which is better than the legal minimum. So your entitlements could differ to those of your colleagues or friends who work for other companies. Check the company maternity policy on your contract of employment. Find out exactly what you might be entitled to by contacting your Human Resources manager, your local Job Centre or Benefits Agency (you will find the telephone number in your local telephone directory).

Health protection

Under UK health and safety legislation, employers must take reasonable measures to protect their employees, and there is a special protection if you are pregnant, have given birth within the last six months or if you are breastfeeding. This might affect you if you are working with hazardous chemicals, or lifting heavy weights, for example.

There are other conditions that might pose a hazard when you are pregnant, such as shocks, vibrations, night work, manual handling of loads and excessive travel. Mental or physical fatigue caused by conditions such as standing for long periods, working at heights, extremes of hot or cold or working with certain biological or chemical agents can also be hazardous. If there is a risk, your employer must either take steps to remove it, or make arrangements so that you are not exposed to it. This could mean either remedying the risk, or, if this cannot be done, temporarily changing your working conditions or offering you suitable alternative work. If that is not possible, you must be suspended on full pay. All employees are entitled to this, regardless of their length of service. Employers should, if possible, provide a suitable place for you to rest when you are pregnant or breastfeeding.

Antenatal appointments

You should be able to take paid time off to attend your antenatal appointments if they take place during working hours. You may be asked to produce evidence that you are pregnant; you will get a Mat B1 form from your doctor or midwife some time after your 20th week of pregnancy. You can use this as proof of your pregnancy and your expected week of childbirth. You should also be able to attend parentcraft or antenatal classes. You have this right regardless of your length of service.

Unfair treatment

You are protected under sex discrimination legislation from being unfairly treated or being dismissed on the grounds of your pregnancy. If you feel that you are being treated unfairly, contact your Trade Union official, ACAS (Advisory, Conciliation and Arbitration Service) or your local Citizen's Advice Bureau.

Maternity leave

All employed mothers have the right to take 26 weeks Ordinary Maternity Leave (OML). If you have worked continuously for your employer for 26 weeks up to and including the 15th week before your baby is due, you will also be eligible for Additional Maternity Leave, which will last for another 26 weeks. Statutory Maternity Pay (SMP) will be paid for 26 weeks.

Those eligible will receive 90 per cent of their salary for the first six weeks, and a fixed amount per week (or 90 per cent of their salary, whichever is lowest) for 20 weeks. This means that you could have up to 52 weeks maternity leave, 26 weeks of which may be paid. Also check the terms in your employment contract as they may be better.

Paternity leave

New fathers are entitled to take one or two weeks leave within eight weeks of their baby's birth, which is paid at the same rate as standard Statutory Maternity Pay. In order to be eligible for this new right, dads must have worked for their employer for at least 26 weeks by the 15th week before their baby is due.

If you are on low pay, you may not be eligible for Statutory Paternity Pay (SPP). Contact your local Job Centre because you may be eligible for Income Support while you're on paternity leave.

Parental leave

Parental leave is unpaid leave of up to thirteen weeks, which can be taken in blocks up to the child's fifth birthday. Each parent is able to take 13 weeks each, as long as they have been employed for at least one year by the time they want to take the leave.

Mothers can take parental leave in addition to any maternity leave. You may need to negotiate the timing of your parental leave with your employer. Parental leave is available to both natural and adoptive parents, and there are also extended periods of leave from work for parents of children who have disabilities.

Childcare

Employees are entitled to short periods of leave to care for dependants. This could be used if childcare arrangements break down, or if a child has been involved in an accident. The leave is not necessarily paid – that is at the discretion of your employer.

JUST THE FACTS
MATERNITY PAY

Your employer may have a maternity policy that you should look at when you find out that you are pregnant. The minimum amount of maternity pay that you can get is outlined below.

- *Statutory Maternity Pay (SMP) is available for up to 26 weeks, for pregnant employees who have worked continuously for the same employer for 26 weeks, ending with the qualifying week, which is the 15th week before the expected week of childbirth. You will need to notify your employer, with the correct amount of notice (see p 114), that you want to apply for this. You must also have average weekly earnings of at least the lower earnings limit for National Insurance Contributions.*

- *Your employer will pay your Statutory Maternity Pay, which is six weeks at 90 per cent of your average gross earnings, and the remainder at the SMP standard rate. This will be paid for 20 weeks. Your HR department will be able to let you know when you need to apply for this.*

- *If you are not eligible for SMP, perhaps because you have just started a new job, or you are self-employed, you may be eligible for Maternity Allowance. This is payable to those who aren't eligible for SMP and who have paid National Insurance contributions for at least 26 weeks out of the 66 weeks ending with the week before the expected week of birth.*

Do I need to start thinking about childcare?

Even if you haven't made any firm decisions about returning to work, it's worth exploring your childcare choices. It is important to start doing your research quite early – certainly during your second trimester – because, unfortunately, the best options are often snapped up very quickly.

What childcare options might be available to me?

Your childcare options are a childminder, nursery, nanny or au pair, although some people ask a relative to care for their child (see p 163). Childminders are registered by the Office for Standards in Education (Ofsted) to care for babies and children in their own home. Many childminders are parents themselves and will also have their own children to care for. Nurseries are childcare centres that employ a combination of qualified

and unqualified staff to care for babies and young children from approximately four months to five years of age in a child-centred environment. A nanny will care for your child or children in your own home. She should hold a recognized qualification in childcare. An au pair is a foreign national who is keen to learn another language and spend some time in a host country. In return for board and lodging with a family, the au pair is expected to do some housework and childcare. Most au pairs are not trained in childcare, and are best employed for older children or where the parent is also at home.

How do I find childcare?

Talk to other parents and parents-to-be. You can also build up your dossier of information by gathering leaflets and brochures about local nurseries, and contacting Childcare Link for information about local childcare or the Children's Information Service (see p 226). Look in the Yellow Pages or on Yell.com for childcare listings of nanny and au pair agencies and nurseries. This will give you a broad picture of prices and availability.

Will I have difficulty finding childcare?

The length of waiting lists varies from place to place, but in urban areas the combination of population density and the legal ratio of three

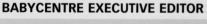

ASK THE EXPERT
ANNA MCGRAIL
BABYCENTRE EXECUTIVE EDITOR

People seem shocked when I say I want to be a full-time mum. Is it the wrong thing to do?

People often react in this way because fewer women choose to be full-time mums these days. Increasingly our society encourages mothers to return to work, and appears not to value mothers who stay at home. The fact that running a home and caring for children is far harder work than many other jobs, with no promotion or financial reward, is often overlooked. Many women find it difficult to make the decision about whether to return to work until their baby arrives. But, when the time comes, only you and your partner can make the decision that's right for you based on your individual circumstances – try not to be influenced by the actions and opinions of others.

BabyCentre Buzz

"I took four months maternity leave with my first son and was ready to return to work when it ended. I enjoy working and don't feel it has hindered my parenting or my children in any way." Amy

"I was sure that I'd be back on the job within three months, but after having my baby, I decided I'd much rather stay at home full time. My partner and I had to make changes to our spending habits, but it's been worth it." Donna

"I went back to work after having my first baby. I think it was good for me to go back because I felt productive making money and accomplishing more. Now that I am about to have my second baby, I'm planning to stay at home. Evenings and weekends are just too short to give my complete attention to both children." Maria

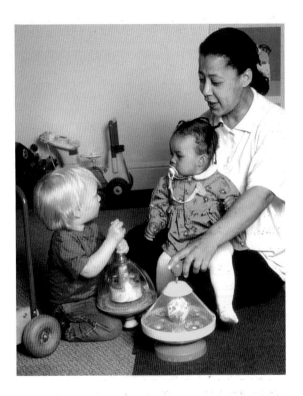

CHILDMINDERS *Childminders usually look after children of mixed age groups. This can closely mirror family life and may help your child feel comfortable around older and younger children. Childminders are usually only allowed to care for one child under the age of one.*

babies to each carer means that the baby rooms in many nurseries could fill their spaces dozens of times over. This is why you must reserve your place as soon as you have made a decision.

If you are looking for a nanny, it may be hard to find someone who is prepared to commit herself to a job before she is ready to hand in her notice to her current employer (usually a minimum of a month beforehand). However, you can start a general search for nanny agencies, begin to interview people, and build up a picture of quality and availability. If you are looking at childminders, you may find that the same principles apply. Many childminders are unwilling to commit themselves too far in advance. Start searching with plenty of time to spare and don't expect to find someone immediately – in fact, it's probably a good idea to see a number of different people and places before making any decision, so you get an idea of the variety in quality, price and style.

Should I consider compromising if I can't get the carer I want?

Yes, finding the carer you want can be difficult and you may have to compromise. Your first choice may be oversubscribed or out of your reach financially. Or you may have your heart set on a nursery place, only to be disappointed in the quality of the local provision. Try to be open to the alternatives. The only thing you should not compromise on is your certainty that your baby will be cared for by the right person or people. Giving yourself a wide time margin to research and apply for a childcare place will increase the possibility of you getting the childcare choice that you want, so that you can rest assured when you return to work.

I'm going on holiday. How can I stay safe now that I'm pregnant?

It's wise to take extra care in the sun when you're pregnant and avoid eating and drinking anything that may cause stomach upsets. However, the main aim is for you to relax and enjoy yourself so try not to worry unnecessarily.

Will flying harm my baby?

No. There is no evidence that recreational flying is harmful to an unborn baby. Heavy exposure to atmospheric radiation during flying has been linked to an increased risk of miscarriage and Down's syndrome and, for this reason, many airlines take the precautionary step of grounding female staff during the first trimester. However, air crew make hundreds of flights and the risk to women who only fly occasionally is negligible.

Is it safe to walk through airport screening machines?

Yes. They use a low-level metal detector, which is considered safe for everyone, including pregnant women. The same holds true for the wands that are passed over passengers. Many people mistakenly think these screening machines take X-rays – they don't. Airport X-ray machines, which emit the same kind of radiation as a dental X-ray, are used only on luggage.

How can I stay comfortable while flying?

Keep your blood circulating by strolling up and down the aisle and doing some simple stretches. When you're sitting, rotate your ankles and wiggle your toes. Wearing support stockings when you fly will help keep your circulation flowing and relieve swollen veins. For maximum protection, put the stockings on before you get out of bed in the morning and keep them on all day. Taking off your shoes may feel nice, but bear in mind that cabin pressure may make your feet swell during the flight and make it difficult for you to put your shoes back on when you land.

How can I be sure my drinking water is safe when I'm travelling abroad?

The best way to ensure your drinking water is safe overseas is to buy bottled water. Avoid tap water unless you're absolutely sure it's safe. Make sure the bottles of water you buy are sealed. In some countries, it is not unknown for people to fill bottles with tap water and sell it as bottled. If you're in any doubt, opt for sparkling water, with a low sodium content if possible. You can also protect yourself against bacteria in the water by boiling it, filtering it or treating it with water purifying tablets. But unless you're on a long camping trip in the middle of nowhere – which is probably highly unlikely – you shouldn't have to go to all that trouble.

QUICK TIP

If you are concerned about the standard of the local water, avoid ice cubes in bars and restaurants. Choose canned or bottled drinks that have been kept cold. If you are self-catering or have a freezer in your room, make your own ice cubes with bottled water.

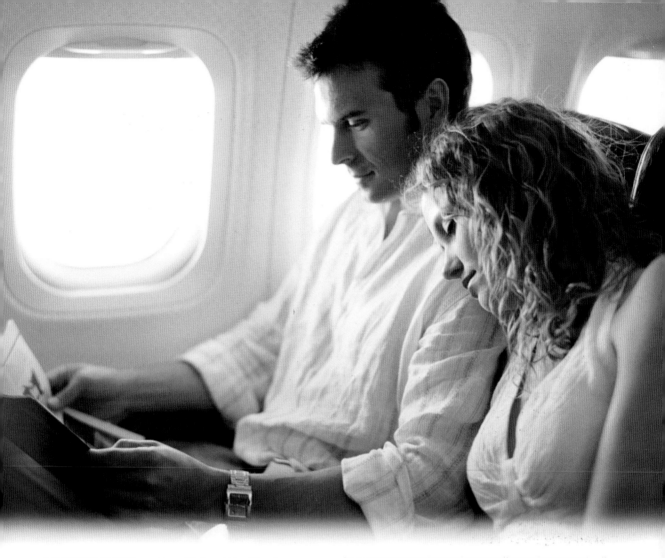

A PLEASANT FLIGHT Request a seat in the middle of the plane over the wing for the smoothest ride, or a bulkhead seat for more legroom. Sitting in an aisle seat will give you more freedom to get up and stretch your legs and go to the toilet.

How can I stay safe in the sun?

Protect your skin with a high factor sunscreen and reapply it regularly. Your skin reacts differently to the sun in pregnancy and exposure to sunlight will intensify your linea nigra and any patches on your face (see p 96). Some pregnant women also find that they are more prone to sunburn, or feel 'prickly' after exposure to the sun. Avoid the midday sun if possible. Wear a sunhat and loose clothes in natural fibres to help you stay cool, and to prevent rubbing and chafing. Carry a fine water spray and hand-held fan, and drink plenty.

JUST THE FACTS
WHAT TO TAKE WITH YOU

If you're going on holiday, take the following:

- *A letter from your doctor or midwife if you are flying in late pregnancy (see p 70), giving your due date and confirming you are fit to fly.*

- *Your maternity notes (see p 84).*

- *Any medication.*

- *Details of your travel insurance.*

- *A European Health Insurance Card (see p 70) if you're travelling in Europe.*

- *Contact details for a local doctor or hospital. In the UK, NHS Direct on 0845 4647 will be able to put you in touch with local services.*

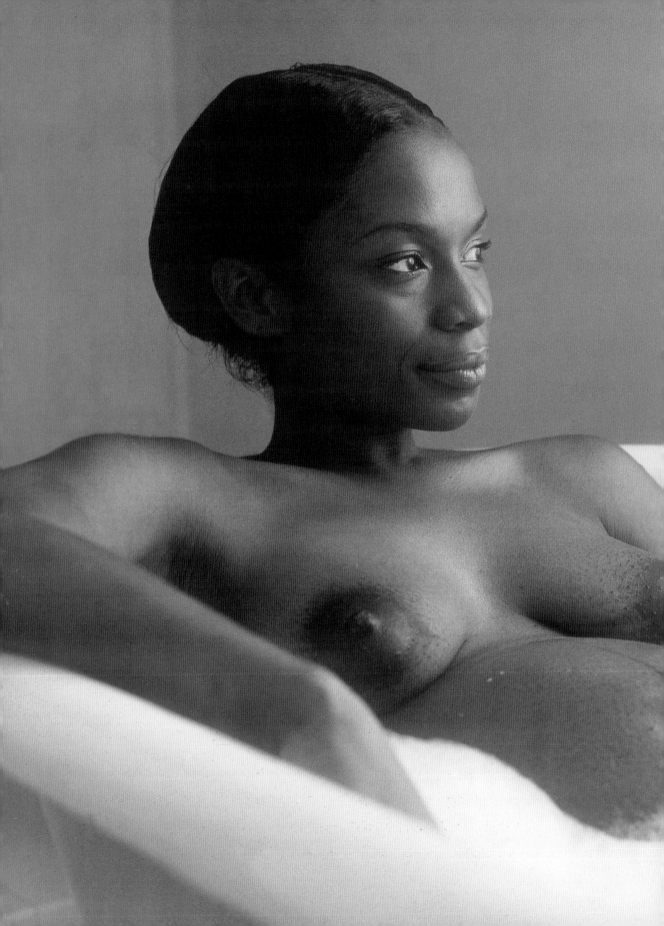

The **third** trimester

28–40 weeks

At last, the end is in sight! These final months may be marked by a mixture of impatience to reach your due date, anxiety about the birth and excitement about meeting your baby. On a practical level, there will be plenty to keep you busy as you prepare for the big day.

28–40 weeks How will my baby develop?

In this final trimester, your baby completes his physical development. As he rapidly gains weight and increases in size, his movements become more restricted. At any time from 36 weeks onwards he will begin his descent into the pelvis, ready to make his journey down the birth canal and into the world.

Your baby at 32 weeks

By now your baby will weigh approximately 2 kg (4 lb) and measure approximately 45 cm (18 in) from head to toe, so he'll be taking up a lot of space in your uterus. Of the weight you are gaining each week, around half will go to your baby. By this stage he has toenails and fingernails and his body and limbs are much more in proportion to the size of his head. His skin is becoming soft and smooth as he plumps up in preparation for the birth. He is beginning to develop real hair, instead of the soft covering of lanugo (see p 78).

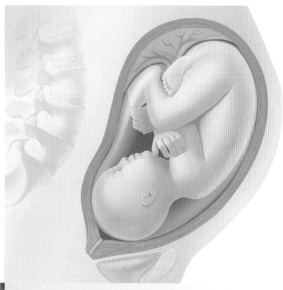

3-D ultrasound scans

Ultrasound technology has improved vastly in the last few years and 3-D scans give an almost photographic reproduction of what your baby will look like. 3-D scans are mainly used to aid the diagnosis of problems such as cleft palate, or give additional information about a known abnormality. A good image of the face can only be obtained if the baby is facing upwards, he does not have his hands in front of his face and there is a good pool of amniotic fluid surrounding the features.

Week 28

Your baby is really starting to grow and fill the available space in your uterus. He now sleeps and wakes at regular intervals. Some experts believe that babies begin to dream by the 28th week of pregnancy but no one knows what it is they dream about. It is known that the brain is active this week – the characteristic grooves start to appear on its surface and more brain tissue develops.

Week 29

Your baby can now open his eyes and will turn his head towards the source of any continuous bright light. Layers of 'white fat' are beginning to form under his skin as he gets ready for his life outside the uterus.

Week 30

Your baby's brain is growing rapidly, and his head is getting bigger to accommodate it. Nearly all babies react to sound by 30 weeks. If you're having a boy, his testicles are moving from their location near the kidneys through the groin. If you're having a girl, her clitoris is relatively prominent because her still small labia don't yet cover it. That will happen in the last few weeks before birth.

Week 31

Your baby's lungs and digestive tract are nearly mature. He continues to open and close his eyes and he can probably see what's going on inside the uterus, distinguish light from dark and even track a light source. If you shine a light on your stomach, your baby may move his head to follow the light or even reach out to touch the moving glow. Some researchers think baring your stomach to light stimulates visual development.

Week 32

Your baby's arms, legs and body continue to fill out – and they are finally proportional in size to his head. He looks more like a newborn now, and weighs about 2 kg (4 lb) and measures about 42 cm (16.7 in) from crown to toe. Your baby's movements are probably changing – they may seem less frequent and less forceful because he's running out of room in your uterus and can't turn any more. He can now move his head from side to side, his organs are continuing to mature and if he was born now he would have an excellent chance of survival.

Week 33

Although his lungs won't be fully developed until just before birth, your baby is inhaling amniotic fluid to exercise his lungs and practise breathing. His central nervous system is also maturing. If your baby is a boy, his testicles have probably moved into his scrotum. Sometimes, one or both testicles doesn't get into position until after the birth, but don't worry. Undescended testicles often correct themselves before the first birthday.

Week 34

The growth spurt continues: by the end of this week your baby could measure as much as 45 cm (17.5 in) long from top to toe. By now, most babies are head down in the uterus (see pp 176–7), although your baby may continue to change position.

Your baby's skull is still quite pliable and not completely joined yet. This is, in part, to enable him to ease out of the relatively narrow birth canal. But the bones in the rest of his body are hardening and his skin is also gradually becoming less red and wrinkled. Most of his basic physical development is now complete.

JUST THE FACTS
YOUR BABY'S THIRD TRIMESTER HIGHLIGHTS

During this trimester, your baby will:

- *Gain approximately 2.25 kg (5 lb) in weight and grow approximately 12.5 cm (5 in).*
- *Usually settles in a head-down position, in preparation for his journey into the world.*

- *Complete all physical development.*
- *Continue forming neurological pathways – the building blocks for learning – in the brain.*
- *Drop down into your pelvis.*

Your baby – ready to be born

At some point in the last few weeks of your pregnancy, your baby will begin his descent into the pelvis – the start of his journey down the birth canal. This process is known as 'engagement' or sometimes as 'lightening'. First babies are more likely to engage earlier, possibly at around 36 weeks, but it doesn't mean the birth is imminent. It is still likely to be several weeks until your baby is born. Second or subsequent babies often don't engage until the final week of pregnancy – and in some instances not until labour begins.

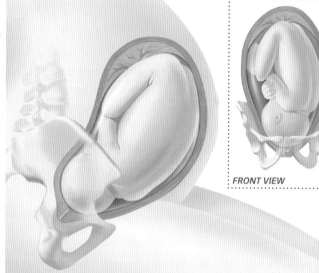

FRONT VIEW

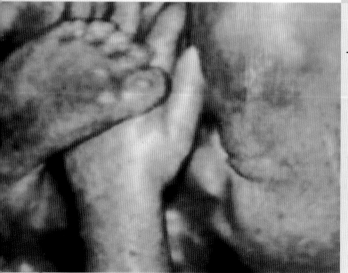

A snug fit

Your baby will rapidly gain weight this trimester. From around the 32nd week to the time he's born, he'll gain approximately a third to a half of his birthweight. As he plumps out, he will gradually begin to move less – there just isn't space to do those somersaults anymore, and there's also less amniotic fluid. You will, however, still be aware of your baby's presence – he'll probably kick and punch to let you know that he's doing okay.

Week 35

Your baby now weighs more than 2.5 kg (5.5 lb). He's filling out and getting rounder – he'll need his fat layers later to regulate his body temperature. If you've been worried about going into labour early, you'll be happy to know that the vast majority of babies delivered at 35 weeks are born healthy and survive without any major problems. Your baby's lungs should be fully developed by now and any breathing problems can be easily treated.

Week 36

Your baby's getting big and is so snug in your womb now that you may notice he isn't moving around as much. You may, however, notice his elbow, foot or head protrude from your stomach when he stretches and squirms about. Soon, as the wall of your uterus and your abdomen stretch thinner and let in more light, your baby will begin to develop daily activity cycles. Your baby now has a fully developed pair of kidneys. His liver can also process some waste products.

Week 37

Congratulations! By the end of this week, your pregnancy will have come full-term – meaning your baby can be born any day now. (Babies born before 37 weeks are premature or pre-term, and those born after 42 weeks are known as post-mature or post-term.) All babies are different but a typical 37-week-old weighs 3 kg (6.5 lb).

Week 38

This week, most of the downy coating of lanugo is shed and the vernix caseosa – the cheese-like coating that covers your baby in the uterus and protects his developing skin – starts to disappear, though some may remain at birth. Your baby swallows both, along with other secretions, and all will stay in her bowels until birth. This blackish mixture, called meconium, will become his first bowel movement.

Week 39

Your baby is now ready to greet the world. At this point, the average full-term newborn is still building a layer of fat to help control body temperature after birth. All your baby's organs are developed and in place, although your baby's lungs will be the last to reach full maturity.

Week 40

The average baby is about 50 cm (20.5 in) long from head to toe and weighs approximately 3.5 kg (7.5 lb) at birth, but anywhere between 2.5 kg (5½ lb) and 4 kg (9 lb) is a healthy range for newborns. The big day is almost here and it won't be long before you're able to cuddle your baby. But don't worry if by the end of this week you're still waiting – only five per cent of babies are born on their expected due date.

Beyond week 40

The big day has come and gone and still no baby. Don't panic! A whopping 75 per cent are born later than their due date. And though it may seem as if your baby is stubbornly refusing to leave the cosy comforts of your uterus, a few studies have found that most overdue babies aren't late at all – their due dates were miscalculated.

If you are still pregnant by the end of week 42, your doctor and midwife will probably suggest inducing labour (see pp 188–9) because after this time your unborn baby is more likely to have problems.

28–40 weeks How will my body change this trimester?

As your baby rapidly gains weight this trimester, you'll begin to feel the strain on your body. Your main priority should be taking care of yourself to help you cope with the symptoms of late pregnancy and prepare you physically and mentally for the birth.

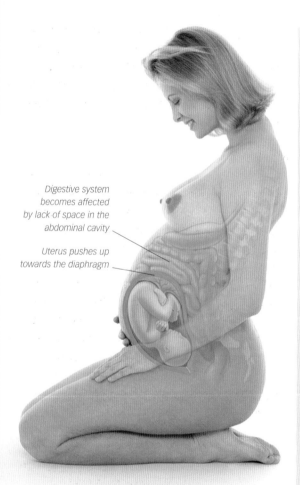

Digestive system becomes affected by lack of space in the abdominal cavity

Uterus pushes up towards the diaphragm

CROWDING OUT *To accommodate your body and your baby's growing needs, your blood volume will have increased by an incredible 40–50 per cent since you first became pregnant. Your uterus will be pushing up near your diaphragm and begin to put pressure on your stomach. The consequences may be shortness of breath and heartburn (see right).*

Your body at 32 weeks

As your developing baby begins to fill out even more of your belly, you'll begin to notice more physical changes. You might begin 'waddling' instead of walking, and finding an easy position to sit in – let alone sleep in – may become more challenging. Using pillows to support your bump (see p 94) and putting your feet up whenever you can may help.

You may have noticed some colostrum ('pre-milk') leaking from your breasts. If so, tuck some nursing pads into your bra to protect your clothes. If your breasts aren't leaking, don't worry. It doesn't happen to all women.

Feeling the strain

Until your baby drops into your pelvis (usually at about 36 weeks for a first pregnancy and later for subsequent pregnancies), you may feel breathless. This happens because your uterus has grown so large it presses up against your diaphragm – the large flat muscle that aids breathing. The crowding of the abdominal cavity can also affect your digestive system, pushing stomach acid upward into the oesophagus and causing heartburn (see p 144), a harmless but uncomfortable condition.

Week 28

If you haven't already signed up for antenatal classes (see pp 132–3), find out if there is a space available now. You're likely to have another antenatal appointment this week and you may have a blood test to check for anaemia, a deficiency of red blood cells. Many pregnant women become mildly anaemic because of normal changes during pregnancy. If your blood group is Rhesus negative and you tested negative for Rh antibodies, you'll have a further test around now (see p 134).

Week 29

Most women gain an average of 5 kg (11 lb) during the third trimester. You may see your midwife more often from now on but you don't have to wait for an appointment. If you want to discuss anything, just phone her. You're probably vacillating between two feelings: 'I've been pregnant forever' and 'Help, I'm not ready for this'. Don't worry, you're not the only one. If you're having your baby in hospital, try to arrange a tour so you know what to expect. Your antenatal class may organize one or the hospital may have an open evening, so ring to check.

Week 30

As your appetite increases to match your baby's third-trimester growth spurt, try to resist eating too many cakes, sweets and fast-food snacks. Make sure you're getting enough iron (see p 98), which helps your baby make red blood cells. If you haven't already adapted your exercise regime, now is a good time to introduce some activities to help your body to stretch and open up ready for the birth. Why not try to find a yoga class specifically for pregnant women (see pp 146–7) – not only will it help you to breathe deeply, but the instructor will show you stretches which may help you get into

and maintain comfortable positions in labour. Even the occasional stretch and wiggle can help you avoid pregnancy niggles such as leg cramps.

Week 31

You've probably gained quite a bit this month – typically 1.4–1.8 kg (3–4 lb). Your baby's demands for nutrients are at their greatest in the final pre-birth growth spurt.

Getting a good night's sleep can become more difficult again in the third trimester. As your bump grows, getting and staying comfortable is harder and you may find pressure on your bladder means midnight trips to the toilet make an unwelcome but necessary return.

Week 32

If you and your partner are getting nervous about the big day, which is very normal, it may help to go over what you learned in your antenatal classes. Think about which pain relief methods you'd be prepared to try and in what order (see pp 172–3). Speak to your midwife for advice if necessary. You could also consider writing a birth plan (see p 166).

You will be advised to stay at home for as long as possible in the early phase of first-stage labour (see pp 178–9). You could use a TENS machine to take the edge off the pain as the strength of the contractions increases – look into hiring one from a local pharmacy or through the internet.

Week 33

If you're concerned that having sex in the final weeks (see pp 152–3) of pregnancy will harm your baby, stop worrying. For most women, sex during pregnancy is fine right up until the time their waters break, and if you happen to go overdue it can even help jumpstart labour.

JUST THE FACTS
YOUR THIRD TRIMESTER HIGHLIGHTS

During this trimester, you will:
- *Start your maternity leave if you are at work.*
- *Attend antenatal classes.*
- *Begin to feel more tired and possibly more anxious as you await labour and birth.*
- *Go for more regular antenatal appointments.*
- *Feel more of a strain on your body, but this will be relieved once your baby engages in your pelvis.*
- *Finally meet your newborn baby!*

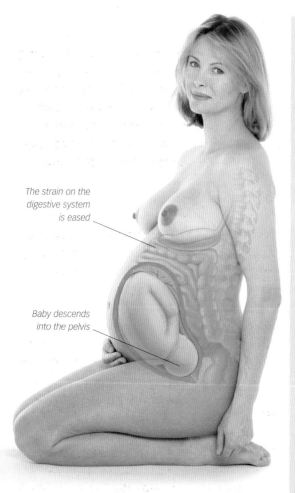

The strain on the digestive system is eased

Baby descends into the pelvis

THE FINAL STAGES *Once your baby has dropped into your pelvis, known as engagement, or lightening, breathing becomes easier but the baby's head may feel heavy between your legs. You may notice an increase in vaginal discharge. If you pass mucus tinged with a tiny amount of blood (see p 141), labour is probably not far away.*

Your body at 40 weeks

Your body has done all the hard work and your baby is likely to have descended into your pelvis (see p 126). The challenge from now on is likely to be more mental than physical as you count the days until your baby is born.

You may find it useful and reassuring to familiarize yourself with the signs of labour (see pp 140–1) and understand the difference between real contractions and practice contractions, known as Braxton Hicks. There is also a possibility that your waters will break, but this doesn't necessarily mean you are in labour.

Clumsiness

Grace and dexterity may disappear altogether in the late weeks of pregnancy. And it's no surprise – you're carrying more weight, your centre of gravity has shifted along with your uterus, and your hips and joints may be looser due to hormones. You're also likely to be distracted by thoughts of the weeks to come. You will be less agile and may be worried about tripping or banging into things, but be reassured that your baby is very well-cushioned by your belly, uterus and the amniotic fluid that surrounds him.

Week 34

You may sleep easier if you start getting prepared for after the birth. Stock up on basics – everything from tins to tights – before shopping becomes too much of a chore. Cook up extra portions to freeze as ready meals for the early weeks – they'll be a godsend. Make a list of important numbers and pin it up by the phone.

Week 35

Lots of women experience pain or twinges in their hips, back or pelvis during the last weeks of pregnancy. Try to avoid any activities that cause pain and see your doctor if it's persistent. You may be referred to a physiotherapist specializing in women's health.

Week 36

You may begin to feel increased pressure in your lower abdomen and notice that your baby is gradually dropping. This lightening or engagement (see p 126) means that your lungs and stomach will finally get a bit more room, so breathing and eating become easier. However, walking may become increasingly uncomfortable – some women even say it feels as if the baby is going to fall out. You may also feel as if you need to pass urine all the time. Practising your pelvic floor exercises (see p 147) can help.

Week 37

Learn to distinguish the true signs of labour (see pp 140–1). Make sure your car always has enough petrol to get you to hospital and that you know the best route and where to park. Finally, now is a good time to get measured for a nursing bra.

Week 38

The next couple of weeks are a waiting game, but try to enjoy this time before the baby arrives. Make sure you eat well and get plenty of rest. Your midwife will drop off a home birth pack about now if you're having your baby at home. Make sure you have packed everything you need if you're having a hospital birth (see pp 166–7).

Week 39

You may be feeling huge and uncomfortable during these final weeks. Try to take it easy – this may be your last opportunity to do so for quite a while. See a film or read a book that has nothing to do with pregnancy or babies. Your partner should try to relax too and enjoy doing all these things as there may not be time for them after the baby arrives.

Week 40

Do you feel that time has flown since the beginning of your pregnancy? Then be prepared: these last few days will probably feel longer than the last nine months!

Beyond 40 weeks

Most doctors and midwives will wait up to another week before considering a pregnancy overdue (see pp 188–9). A pregnancy is considered post-mature when it goes past 42 weeks. Talk through your options with your antenatal teacher or midwife if you don't go into labour on your own.

Your midwife or doctor may suggest methods to try to get labour started naturally (see pp 188–9). It can be hard to cope with the waiting now you are overdue. If people are phoning to ask if you've had the baby yet and you're sick of repeating yourself, put a message on your answering machine.

Should I attend antenatal classes?

Most women find antenatal classes a useful source of information, especially if it's their first pregnancy. Hospital classes, run by midwives, are free, but you may have to book and pay for other types of classes. It's advisable to sign up early to avoid disappointment as many classes get booked up quickly.

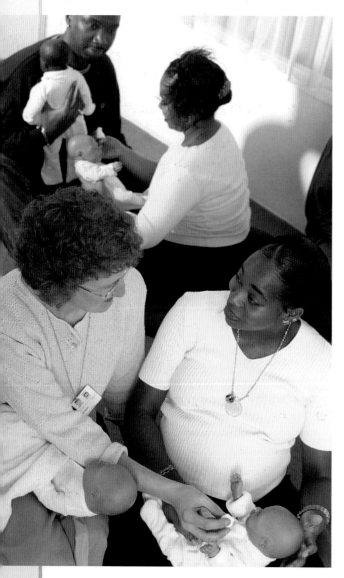

What are antenatal classes?

Antenatal classes come in various forms, but all have the same aim – to help prepare you for labour, birth and parenthood. Those run by midwives or your local hospital are free, but you may have to pay for other types, such as National Childbirth Trust (NCT) (see p 228) and Active Birth Centre classes (see p 226). You may find it helpful to go to more than one type of class. When attending classes other than those run by a hospital or health centre, check the teacher has been properly trained.

What are NCT classes?

NCT classes are run by the National Childbirth Trust (see p 228) and taught by highly trained teachers. As well as going over the topics covered in the free classes, they prepare you to make informed choices about labour and birth.

I don't have a partner. Is there a class that's suitable for me?

Yes, you could try women-only classes. Single women and those whose partners are away may find these classes particularly useful. Many others

BABYCARE SKILLS *As well as preparing you for labour and birth, antenatal classes teach you some of the basic techniques for looking after your newborn baby.*

JUST THE FACTS
WHAT YOU'LL LEARN AT ANTENATAL CLASSES

Antenatal classes help you to focus on your pregnancy and forthcoming birth, but they are also a great place to meet other parents-to-be. The content of the classes will vary, but should include information about the following:

- *The process of labour and childbirth.*
- *Details of medical procedures and interventions.*
- *The latest research suggestions about possible physical preparations for labour and childbirth.*
- *Advice on relaxation techniques.*
- *The opportunity to learn about and experiment with different birth positions.*
- *A guide to pain relief.*
- *The chance to learn and try out massage skills and breathing techniques.*
- *The time to ask questions and rehearse the possible decisions you may have to make during the course of your labour.*
- *An idea of what to expect immediately after the birth and in the first few weeks of parenthood.*

also enjoy the close bond that can develop in women-only classes, where you often have the opportunity to talk and discuss subjects that may not be covered during couples' classes.

My partner thinks he'll be the only man at the class. How can I encourage him?

Find out about couples' classes. These are usually for first-time parents and help both partners get involved in the preparations for labour and birth. For many men, going to a class gives them a specific time to focus on the pregnancy. It's also an opportunity to meet other fathers-to-be. Often men have had no chance to talk about the pregnancy and find the classes give them this opportunity.

This is my second pregnancy, so do I need to attend classes?

You could consider going to refresher classes. These are aimed at women who already have children and sometimes crèche facilities are offered. Most antenatal classes are 'client-led' to a greater or lesser extent, but this is especially true of refresher classes. For example, second-time mothers often want to talk about their birth experiences and to be updated on research and changes in birth practices, but may feel totally confident about feeding their babies. If this is the case, issues such as bottle-feeding versus breastfeeding may not be discussed.

Will I be offered a hospital tour?

From about 34 weeks onwards, you may be offered a session at the hospital which will include a tour round the labour ward. This gives parents the chance to become familiar with the layout and to look at the facilities available, for example, a birthing pool. Some hospitals (especially if they are short-staffed) are now offering a virtual tour on CD.

How are active birth classes different to normal classes?

The emphasis tends to be on positive physical preparation and active participation in the birth. Contact the Active Birth Centre (see p 226) for a list of teachers in your area or find out where they are available from other mums-to-be.

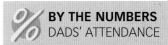

BY THE NUMBERS
DADS' ATTENDANCE

Will your partner be preparing for the birth of your child with you through books and antenatal classes?

72% Yes, he's very keen.

16% No, I fill him in afterwards.

12% No, he doesn't have time.

Source: Based on a BabyCentre. co.uk poll of 2,298 women.

Will I be offered more tests this trimester?

You will attend antenatal appointments roughly every two weeks this trimester. If your pregnancy is straightforward, you're unlikely to be offered more tests. Your midwife will check your progress and your baby's development, and only request further tests to be carried out if she has particular concerns.

Will I have any more ultrasound scans?

You're unlikely to need an ultrasound scan in late pregnancy, unless you are having twins, your previous baby was small, or you have a complication such as diabetes or high blood pressure. Your midwife might recommend one if she's unsure of your baby's position (see pp 176–7). A scan might also be recommended if there is any concern about how your baby is thriving and to measure the level of amniotic fluid. If your placenta was low, it will be checked again at 36 weeks.

ASK THE EXPERT
CHRISSIE HAMMONDS
MIDWIFE SONOGRAPHER

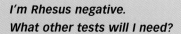

I'm Rhesus negative.
What other tests will I need?

It's now recommended that Rhesus negative women have a blood test at 28 weeks. You should also be offered injections of anti-D immunoglobulin (anti-D) at 28 and 34 weeks to prevent your immune system from reacting to any of your baby's cells. Sometimes an anti-D injection is given in situations that could lead to your baby's blood mixing with yours, such as a hard blow to the stomach, chorionic villus sampling (see p 37), amniocentesis (see p 86), a termination or an ectopic pregnancy (see p 18). You should also be given anti-D if you have an external cephalic version (see p 177) or have any vaginal bleeding or a miscarriage after 12 weeks of pregnancy.

What is Doppler sonography?

This is a non-invasive test that can be done at the same time as an ultrasound. It uses the same equipment to measure blood flow in different parts of your own or your baby's body. You may have one if, for example, your midwife is concerned about the working of your placenta and whether your baby is growing enough. In this case she can arrange for a growth scan where Doppler sonography will be used to evaluate the flow of blood in the umbilical cord or in your baby's body itself. This will reveal whether your baby needs to be delivered early or other measures are needed to protect his health.

Should I monitor my baby's movements?

Not so long ago, women were advised to monitor their baby's movements with a fetal kick chart, on which they noted the number of times their baby had moved by roughly the same time each day. But these charts are used less and less now as they were easy to forget about, and the kick patterns didn't always match up, which caused unnecessary concern among women. Women are usually advised to get used to their baby's pattern during waking hours and inform their midwife if they think there is a change in that pattern. If you are concentrating on something else, you may not have noticed your baby's movements. If you want some reassurance, encourage your baby to move: either lie down on

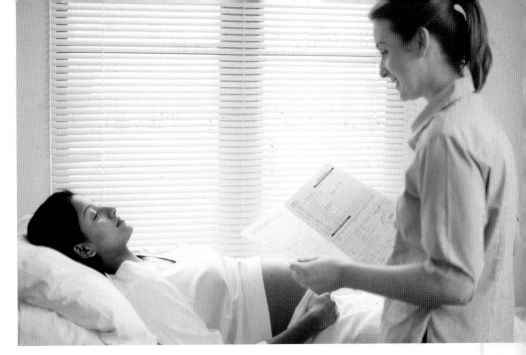

FINAL CHECKS Your midwife will begin antenatal appointments by asking you how you are feeling and answer any of your concerns. She will carry out a physical examination to check your baby's size and position in the uterus.

your side (with support under your bump) and stay still or just put your feet up and relax. Playing music to your stomach may also encourage your baby to move.

Why do I need a glucose tolerance test?

This test is recommended if there is too much sugar in your urine, which may be a sign of gestational diabetes. This condition can lead to the baby being very large. Before the test you will be asked not to eat anything for six hours. You will then attend a special clinic where the test will be carried out.

On arrival, a nurse will take a blood sample from you. If you are nervous about giving blood, ask a friend to stay with you. The first blood sample is used to measure the level of sugar in your blood when you have been fasting and is called a baseline test. You will next be asked to drink a very sweet, sugary mixture and your blood will then be tested at set intervals and the measurements compared with the normal range. It's reassuring to remember that most women who have sugar in their urine at their antenatal appointment turn out to have normal blood sugar levels in the glucose tolerance test.

I've been told I have protein in my urine. What does this mean?

The presence of protein in your urine gives information about how your kidneys are working. Small amounts of protein are not uncommon, and may simply mean that your kidneys are working harder than before pregnancy. Your body may be fighting a minor infection, and the midwife may send your urine sample for analysis, to establish whether you have a urine infection. You may then be prescribed antibiotics. At your next appointment the midwife will establish whether there is still protein present, and whether the amount has increased, which may be an indication of pre-eclampsia (see below). If your urine sample has high levels of protein, a blood sample may also be taken to check for pre-eclampsia.

What is pre-eclampsia?

This is a potentially serious condition that can affect the health of both you and your unborn baby. Signs are raised blood pressure, increased protein in the urine and swelling of fingers, feet and face. Always seek medical advice immediately if you notice any abnormal swelling.

What symptoms am I likely to experience in the last trimester?

After the relative bliss of mid-pregnancy, you may find yourself having to deal with unwanted symptoms in the final months. As well as the physical effects brought on by your increased size, pregnancy may begin to play havoc with your memory.

I often feel breathless. Should I be worried about this?

No, this is a normal symptom of late pregnancy. Many women find they go through a breathless phase, often between about 28–36 weeks. This is the time when your internal organs are being pushed up by your growing baby. There's just not enough room for you to take a deep breath. At around 36 weeks your baby begins to settle down into the pelvis ready for the birth, and this relieves the pressure so breathing becomes easier. If you're asthmatic, discuss your condition with your doctor or midwife. Rest assured that you're not depriving your baby of oxygen. Your respiratory system adapts during pregnancy so your body can process oxygen more efficiently.

I've become very clumsy. Is this normal?

Yes, and it should come as no surprise if you consider what your body's going through: you're carrying more weight, your centre of gravity has changed with your growing uterus, and your fingers, toes, and other joints are all loosening due to pregnancy hormones. Tripping and falling is a huge fear among pregnant women, but remember that your baby is well protected by the bony pelvis and the waters that she floats around in. If you do fall, contact your doctor or midwife just to make sure everything is alright. Try not to put yourself in situations where you have a high risk of falling (like dancing on a crowded floor). Watch out for wet, icy, or uneven surfaces when walking and don't carry anything that you can't safely drop. Clumsiness is only a temporary, pregnancy-related condition. If your clumsiness is accompanied by dizziness, headaches, blurred vision or any pain, contact your doctor or midwife immediately.

Why do I keep forgetting everything?

You're probably just overwhelmed by the huge life changes you're about to experience. Those concerns can crowd the mind of an otherwise

BabyCentre Buzz

"I've never been a clumsy person, but in these final weeks of pregnancy I've started dropping glasses. If there's a glass in the house, I manage to drop or crack it nine times out of ten. My husband finally bought a set of plastic tumblers. He says if I keep using real glasses, we won't have any left by the time the baby is born!" Andrea

"For some reason, I've lost all sense of spatial awareness, which has really affected my ability to parallel park. After bumping into the cars behind and in front of me, inadvertently honking my car horn in the process, I've now decided I'd rather pay to use a car park." Erica

clear-headed person. Try devising strategies to help remember what's important and reduce frustration. Carry a small notebook in which you can jot down reminders, keep a detailed daily calendar and put items you use often such as keys, in the same place. Forgetfulness may be your cue to try simplifying your life so make some time to relax.

I seem to spend most of my time in the loo! What can I do?

In the last trimester your growing baby tends to squash your bladder; it can be up to a third smaller than before pregnancy. Even when your bladder is empty, the pressure on it can make it feel full. Also, pregnant women sometimes have trouble emptying their bladder completely, so lean forward to ensure it is empty. Try drinking almost nothing for the hour or two before bedtime to cut down on night-time trips, but keep drinking at least 8–10 glasses of water each day. Some say it's nature's cruel way of training you for the many nights of interrupted sleep once your baby arrives! Talk to your doctor or midwife if you feel pain or burning when you urinate as a urinary infection can lead to a kidney infection and increase the risk of premature labour.

How can I prevent varicose veins?

Raise your feet and legs whenever possible: if you sit at a desk, keep a stool or box underneath. Before getting out of bed, put on special support tights. By putting them on before standing, you'll prevent excess blood from gathering in your legs. If you have to stand for long periods, stimulate circulation by going up on your tip-toes several times. Don't cross your legs when seated.

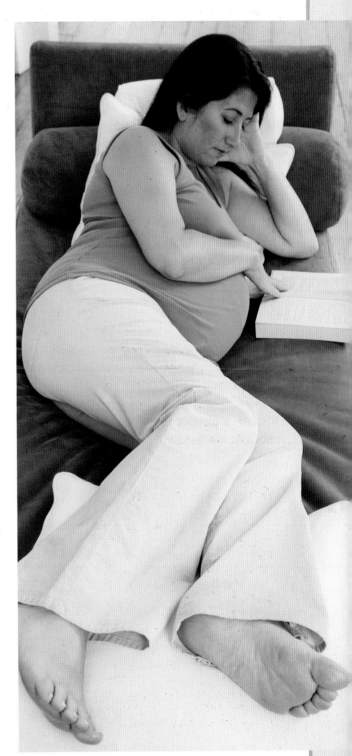

EASING THE STRAIN Lying down on your left side with your feet elevated on a pillow helps the veins in your legs do their work and reduces the likelihood of getting varicose veins.

How can I relax and relieve stress?

Just because you're expecting a baby doesn't mean the rest of your life has stopped. Many pregnant women, especially those who are in full-time work or who already have children, find they still have to manage the stresses and strains of everyday life, in addition to making preparations for their baby's arrival.

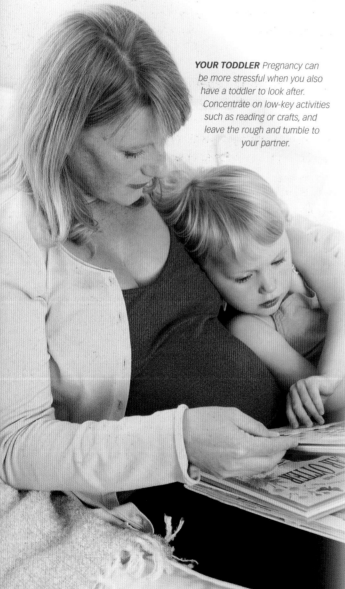

YOUR TODDLER *Pregnancy can be more stressful when you also have a toddler to look after. Concentrate on low-key activities such as reading or crafts, and leave the rough and tumble to your partner.*

I'm feeling stressed. Is this normal?

Yes, lots of pregnant women suffer from stress. As well as concerns about your unborn baby's health and wellbeing, you may be thinking about the impending labour, wondering how you'll manage after the birth and whether you have bought everything you need. Whatever it is that's worrying you, it's important to try to de-stress. There are many positive steps you can take to overcome these feelings (see right).

Will stress harm my unborn baby?

Isolated periods of stress experienced from time to time will have no harmful effect on you or your baby. Some studies have suggested that prolonged, severe stress in early pregnancy can increase your chances of pregnancy complications, such as pre-eclampsia (see p 135) and premature birth, and some have shown a link to hyperactive disorders in pre-school children. It is important to seek help if you are finding stress a problem.

Why do I feel so guilty for putting my feet up?

It's a simple thing, but sometimes so difficult to take time out for yourself. Not only is this good for you, but also extremely good for your baby – so don't feel guilty about 'doing nothing'. Obviously, if you have a child already it can be hard to find the time to rest, so if possible make it a priority to get help with childcare whenever you can, while you have a well-earned break.

What complementary therapies can I try to help me relax?

Massage in pregnancy is a fantastic way to de-stress. The Active Birth Centre (see p 226) runs a pregnancy and labour massage course for partners and there are lots of massage books available with tips and advice for pregnant women. If you are using essential oils, it's important to make sure they are safe for use in pregnancy. Oils safe for use after 20 weeks include most lavender oils, citrus oils and ylang ylang, but you should check with a qualified aromatherapist. Reflexology is also a lovely way to relax, but make sure the therapist is qualified in working with pregnant women.

Some mums-to-be find that Bach Flower Remedies, available from health-food shops, can help to ease stress, particularly Walnut Remedy and Rescue Remedy. Meditation and positive visualization techniques can also help. Meditation is a way of relaxing by concentrating on a mental focus, and positive visualization is a technique for releasing anxieties by creating an inner picture of a peaceful scene. Buy some relaxation tapes to play – they are great for helping your mind switch off.

I'm finding my journey to work so stressful. What can I do?

Like a lot of women, you may plan on working until just a few weeks before your due date because you want more time after your baby is born. Ask your employer if you can avoid rush hours, particularly if you use public transport. Perhaps starting work earlier and finishing earlier would be possible, or even working from home one or two days a week.

Make sure you always sit down while travelling and if you are not offered a seat, ask for one. Try not to feel embarrassed – most people are more than willing to give up their seats if asked, but are often not sure if they should offer.

QUICK TIP

Pamper yourself: treat yourself to a spa that offers treatments for pregnant women. Pregnancy is also the perfect time to treat yourself to beauty treatments you never normally splash out on. When your bump gets too big for you to cut your toenails, have a pedicure.

Is it possible to relieve stress by adapting my diet and exercising?

Yes, eating calming nutrients can help suppress the hormones that rise at times of stress. Foods containing B vitamins, such as yeast extract and wholegrain foods, increase your levels of the anti-stress hormone serotonin.

Exercise also helps to relieve stress. If you're in any doubt about what exercises you can do during pregnancy, check with your midwife. If you attend exercise classes, always tell your teacher that you are pregnant. Swimming (see p 146) is the perfect exercise for pregnancy as it keeps you toned and healthy, without being too hard on your joints. Aquanatal classes for pregnant women are also a fun way of keeping fit.

IF YOU DO NOTHING ELSE...

- *Put yourself first for once and don't feel guilty.*
- *Be nice to yourself – you deserve it.*
- *Stay positive and list all the things you're looking forward to about your baby's arrival.*

How will I know if I'm in labour?

Labour is different for every woman, and pinpointing when it begins is not really possible. It's more of a process than a single event, when a number of physiological changes in your body work together to help deliver a baby. Try to familiarize yourself with the main signs and always seek advice from your midwife or doctor if necessary.

Can I still call my midwife, even if I'm not entirely sure I'm in labour?

Yes. Doctors and midwives are used to getting phone calls from women who are uncertain if they're in labour. They will want to know the timing of your contractions, whether you can talk through a contraction and whether your waters have broken. You should also let them know if your baby is moving less, if you have any vaginal bleeding, fever, severe headaches, changes in your vision or persistent (rather than intermittent) abdominal pain.

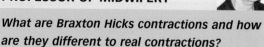

ASK THE EXPERT
LESLEY PAGE
PROFESSOR OF MIDWIFERY

What are Braxton Hicks contractions and how are they different to real contractions?

Towards the middle of your pregnancy, you may notice the muscles of your uterus tightening for anywhere from 30 to 60 seconds. Not all women feel these random, usually painless contractions, which get their name from John Braxton Hicks, an English doctor who first described them in 1872. Doctors and midwives believe that Braxton Hicks contractions are part of your body getting ready for labour. Real contractions are noticeably longer, more regular, frequent and painful than Braxton Hicks contractions. Also, labour pains will increase in frequency, duration, and intensity as time goes on, whereas Braxton Hicks contractions remain unpredictable and without a regular rhythm.

What should I do if my waters break?

First, don't panic! Put on a sanitary towel – this will also make it easier to see the colour of the fluid you are losing. The amount of fluid you lose may vary from a slight trickle to a large gush. Amniotic fluid is almost clear with a yellow tinge, and possibly a little bloodstained to begin with. By the end of pregnancy, there can be nearly 1 litre (1.5 pt) fluid, so it can be quite a shock if your waters do come out in a big gush.

If there is a lot of fluid, a sanitary pad will not be adequate and an old hand towel – while undignified – is more practical, especially if you need to travel by car to hospital. If it is a small trickle every now and again, it is important to make sure it is not leakage of urine, which can also happen in late pregnancy.

Regardless of how many weeks pregnant you are when your waters break, you should be seen fairly quickly for an assessment. Once your waters have broken, there is less protection against getting an infection. Some hospitals will admit you to the delivery ward, while others may see you in the antenatal clinic.

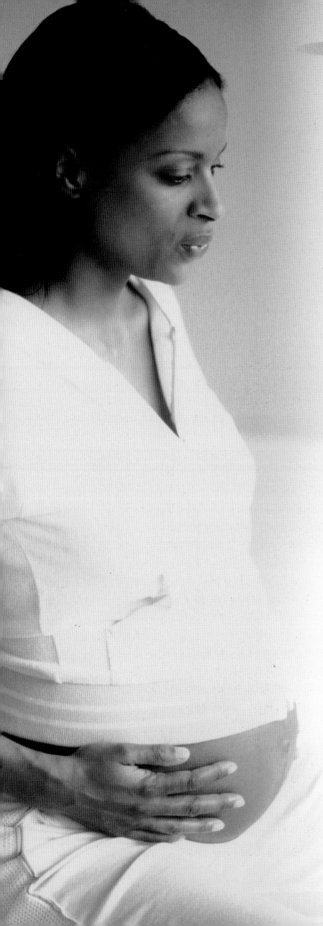

What should I do to take care of myself in early labour?

It's very important to drink plenty of fluids. Some women want to eat at this stage, but avoid anything too heavy on your stomach. Try taking a warm bath or shower to ease any aches and pains. Leaning forward and having your back massaged may help ease pain. And if you can, try to get some rest to prepare you for the hard work ahead.

Can I have contractions and not actually be in labour?

Yes. You're in false labour if your cervix doesn't dilate (your doctor or midwife can confirm this during an examination), contractions are erratic and don't feel increasingly intense, and any abdominal or back pain is easily relieved by a bath or massage.

JUST THE FACTS
THE SIGNS OF LABOUR

These are the four signs of labour:

- *Contractions occur at regular and increasingly shorter intervals and become longer and stronger in intensity.*

- *You may have persistent lower back pain, and possibly a cramped premenstrual feeling.*

- *You may notice the appearance of a bloody show (a brownish or blood-tinged discharge). This is the mucus plug that blocks the cervix, and labour could be imminent – or it could be several days away. Still, it's a sign that things are moving along.*

- *Your cervix will become progressively thinner, softer (this process is called effacement) and dilated – up to 10 cm.*

Note: If your waters break, you are not necessarily in labour (see left).

Premature labour and birth

In medical terms, a premature birth is when a baby arrives before 37 completed weeks of pregnancy. It is still very difficult for doctors to predict whether a woman will go into labour prematurely, but there are known risk factors. Technological developments have meant the outlook for babies born prematurely has greatly improved.

Coping with premature labour

It's probably hard to describe the shock of finding out that you are going to give birth several weeks, or even months, earlier than you had anticipated. You will naturally feel very worried, and perhaps out of control because of all the medical attention you are receiving. Do ask your midwives and doctors to explain everything to you.

Hospital tests

You will be given a vaginal examination to see whether your cervix is shortening and opening. A number of tests may be carried out to check for infection. Another test is for a substance called fetal fibronectin in your amniotic fluid, which can indicate that your baby will be born soon.

Monitoring

If your doctors are not certain whether you are in labour, you will be admitted to the antenatal ward for observation. Doctors can't stop labour if it's really underway and resting won't help either. However, if you are less than 34 weeks pregnant, your doctors can offer you a drug to delay the birth so that there is time to transfer you to a hospital with an Intensive Care Baby Unit.

You will also be offered steroid drugs to help your baby's lungs mature. A baby's lungs may not be ready to breathe air until about 36 weeks of pregnancy, so a baby born before then may have breathing difficulties. Steroid injections help his lungs to mature more quickly. If you are more than 34 weeks pregnant, your doctors will probably allow labour to continue. Your baby's heartbeat will be monitored throughout labour.

Your baby's health

The health of the baby usually depends on the level of prematurity:

- A baby born after 34 weeks is unlikely to have any serious problems, although he may be a bit small and may have some breathing difficulties.
- Babies born earlier than this still have a lot of growing to do and their internal organs need to mature. They may be quite weak and find sucking and breathing difficult.
- Babies born as early as 22–25 weeks now stand a chance of survival, but more than half will have disabilities ranging from mild to severe.

Caring for your baby

You can still help to care for your baby by changing his nappy, stroking him, talking to him and perhaps holding him. You can express your breast milk to be fed to him. Remember that he needs the special comfort that only his parents can give him.

YOUR PREMATURE BABY If your baby is born before 34 weeks, he may need to go immediately to the Special Care or Intensive Care Baby Unit. A baby born between 34 and 37 weeks may not need any medical treatment. He may be able to go straight to the postnatal ward with you or be admitted with you to a special ward where there is a high ratio of staff to mothers.

The following increase the risk of premature birth:

- Infections of the vagina and urinary tract.

- Expecting more than one baby.

- Smoking or using recreational drugs.

- Living in poverty.

- Being the victim of domestic violence.

- Some abnormalities of the uterus.

- Previous surgery to the cervix.

- Previous abortion or previous miscarriages, especially at 16–24 weeks.

- Previous premature birth.

- Change of partner between your first two babies; it increases your risk of pre-eclampsia (see p 135).

How can I relieve digestive problems?

A combination of pregnancy hormones and the crowding-out of your internal organs as your baby grows may cause havoc with your digestive system, leading to problems such as heartburn and constipation. However, there are simple remedies, such as adapting your diet, to minimize the problem.

Recently I've felt a terrible burning sensation after eating. Is it heartburn?

Probably. Many women experience heartburn for the first time during pregnancy – and although it's common and harmless, it can be uncomfortable and painful. Heartburn is a burning sensation that often extends from the lower throat to the bottom of

Crowded abdominal cavity

Uterus grows

the breastbone. It is caused by both hormonal and physical changes in your body. During pregnancy, the placenta produces the hormone progesterone, which relaxes the smooth muscles of the uterus. This hormone also relaxes the valve that separates the oesophagus from the stomach, allowing gastric acids to seep back up the pipe, which causes that uncomfortable sensation of heartburn.

Progesterone also slows down the wave-like contractions of the stomach, making digestion sluggish. In later pregnancy, your growing baby crowds your abdominal cavity, slowing elimination and pushing up the stomach acids to cause heartburn. Many women start getting heartburn and indigestion in the second half of their pregnancy. And – unfortunately – it usually comes and goes until your baby is born.

Why am I so constipated, and should I be concerned about it?

Constipation is a common problem in pregnancy, affecting at least half of all pregnant women. The culprits are the pressure of your growing uterus on your rectum, along with pregnancy hormones, which slow the transit of food through

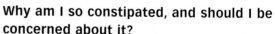

ACID ATTACK As your abdomen becomes more crowded, from mid-pregnancy onwards, stomach acid may be pushed up into the oesophagus and cause heartburn.

your digestive tract. Constipation is more of an inconvenience than a major problem for most women, but if it persists, do mention it to your doctor. Sometimes, constipation can lead to haemorrhoids or piles (see right), which can be extremely uncomfortable. But these can be treated, and both conditions should resolve themselves fairly soon after your baby is born.

What can I do to relieve constipation?

Some iron pills can make constipation worse so ask your midwife or doctor whether it makes sense to switch to a different type of supplement. Eat high-fibre foods such as cereals, whole-grain breads and fresh fruits and vegetables every day. Drink plenty of water or fruit juice – at least 8–10 glasses a day is the recommendation. Prune juice might also be helpful. Exercise can help to ease constipation, and leave you feeling more fit and healthy. Don't take over-the-counter laxatives without seeking medical advice because they can leave you dehydrated.

QUICK TIP

Some women who have piles find comfort with an ice pack, while others swear by warmth. Alternate between warm baths and cold ice packs to find which brings you the most relief.

What cause piles during pregnancy?

Pregnancy makes women more prone to piles, varicose veins (see p 137) and even bleeding gums because when you're pregnant, your blood volume increases and your blood vessels stretch more easily. This may cause your blood vessels to become dilated. In particular, the veins below the level of your uterus are more susceptible to becoming varicose – abnormally swollen or dilated – as the uterus places increased pressure on them. Constipation (see left), which often accompanies pregnancy, can also cause or aggravate piles.

Piles sound dreadful! How can I avoid getting them?

Although you're more susceptible to piles when pregnant, they're not inevitable. It helps to go to the loo as soon as you have the urge to have a bowel movement, and don't linger on the toilet. But the most effective way to avoid piles is to eat a high-fibre diet, drink plenty of water, and try to get some regular exercise, even if it's only a short walk. You can also ask your doctor or midwife about using a stool softener. Doing pelvic floor exercises (see p 105) can also help.

JUST THE FACTS
HOW TO MINIMIZE HEARTBURN

Seek medical advice if none of the following suggestions eliminate your heartburn:

- *Limit your intake of rich or spicy dishes, chocolate, citrus fruits, alcohol and coffee.*

- *Eat small, frequent meals, take small mouthfuls and chew your food well.*

- *Avoid drinking large quantities of fluids during meals. It's important to drink 8–10 glasses of water daily, but drink it between meals.*

- *Try not to lie down for at least an hour after eating. The valve between your stomach and oesophagus is more lax than usual due to the relaxant effects of pregnancy hormones. You can get stomach acid in your oesophagus if you lie down too soon after eating.*

- *Sleep propped up with several pillows or elevate the head of your bed. Gravity will help keep your stomach acids where they should be.*

- *An over-the-counter antacid that contains magnesium or calcium may ease discomfort, but check with your doctor before taking one.*

How can I stay active in late pregnancy?

Exercise becomes more of a challenge in the third trimester, but it also offers some welcome rewards. A moderate, gentle exercise routine can be a great way to keep common pregnancy discomforts at bay, improve your body image and calm any anxiety you may be experiencing as your due date approaches.

Is it true that swimming is the best exercise for late pregnancy?

Most women like swimming in late pregnancy because being bouyant in the water makes them feel almost weightless. Swimming also improves circulation, increases muscle tone and strength and builds endurance. The water supports your joints and ligaments as you exercise, preventing injury, and protects you from overheating. Swimming can also help with swelling and the discomfort caused by varicose veins in your legs or vulval area. Always start slowly, warm up and cool down gradually, and don't over-exert yourself or exercise too hard. All you need to do is stay fit, so take it easy. Alternating breaststroke with floating on your back and gently kicking your legs will give you a good all-round workout. Avoid breaststroke if you have pain in your back or at the front of your pelvis. A maternity swimsuit may be more comfortable now that you're well into your pregnancy. You might also want to find an aquanatal exercise class offered by a qualified instructor.

JUST THE FACTS
DANGER SIGNS

Stop exercising and seek medical advice if you have any of the following:

- Vaginal bleeding.
- Blurred vision.
- Nausea.
- Dizziness or fainting.
- Breathlessness.
- Heart palpitations.
- Swelling in the hands, feet and ankles.
- Sharp pain in the abdomen or chest.
- Sudden change in body temperature.
- Leaking of amniotic fluid.
- Contractions that don't subside with rest.

How will I benefit from yoga classes?

Yoga, when combined with a cardiovascular exercise such as walking, can be an ideal way to maintain fitness when you're pregnant. When you stretch or do yoga, you're toning your muscles and limbering up with little, if any, impact on your joints. It's good to practise yoga in the third trimester in preparation for the birth. It is beneficial because it helps you breathe and relax, which in turn can help you adjust to the physical demands of labour. Yoga training will help you fight the urge to tighten up when you're in pain, and show you how to breathe, instead. As with any other exercise, you need to take certain precautions. Never attempt upside-down poses while you're pregnant and avoid any movements that require you to be flat on your back – this decreases blood-flow to the uterus. Never

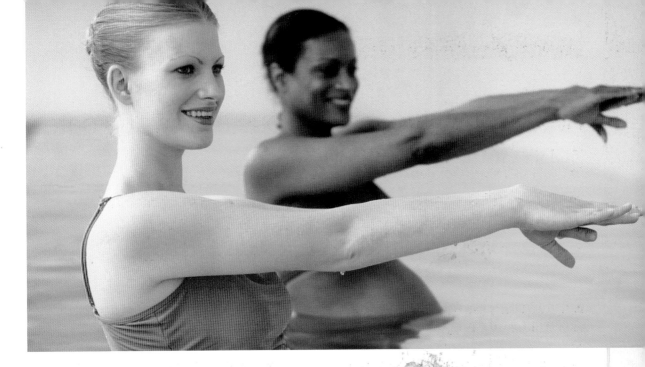

AQUANATAL CLASSES Exercising while standing in water is gentler on your joints and can help lessen swelling in the legs, which is a common symptom of late pregnancy.

force or strain during any pose or stretch, especially during movements that stretch the abdominal muscles. You are more apt to tear and strain muscles now because the pregnancy hormone relaxin, which allows the uterus to expand, also acts on other connective tissue. If you experience pain in the back, hips or pelvis, modify your postures. Always find a specialist pregnancy yoga class.

Is Pilates a good exercise for pregnancy?

Yes, because it targets the tummy and pelvic floor muscles, which can weaken during pregnancy. Many Pilates exercises are performed in a hands and knees position, and this is ideal for pregnancy. It helps to take the stress off your back and pelvis, and towards the end of your pregnancy can help to position your baby ready for delivery. Before trying Pilates, ensure you can perform a strong pelvic floor contraction by squeezing in your pelvic floor muscles and holding them for at least 10 seconds. If you cannot maintain a 'stable core' by tightening your pelvic floor and lower abdominal muscles then you risk overstressing your joints and ligaments.

Positions that involve lying on your tummy or back are not appropriate for mid-pregnancy and beyond. Find a Pilates class designed for pregnant women.

What exercises help to prepare for birth?

Squats strengthen the legs, giving you the ability and stamina to use this position during the birth. Keep your back straight while squatting and hold onto something if necessary. Exercises on your hands and knees help the baby to get into a good position for delivery. Focusing on the relaxation part of pelvic floor exercises can help to prepare for the crowning or appearance of your baby's head.

BabyCentre Buzz

"I'm doing yoga and walking most days. This pregnancy has gone smoother than my first, and I attribute that to staying in shape." Karen

"Since going swimming three times a week, I've been sleeping better and my back pain has improved." Tina

"I'm in week 36 and my only relief is swimming. It eases the pain in my varicose veins. I'd happily sleep in the pool!" Libby

I'm beginning to feel anxious as my due date approaches. Is this normal?

Most women experience some anxiety about labour and birth, especially if it's their first baby. Try to maintain a positive attitude without being locked into specific expectations. Talking to your midwife may help to alleviate some of your fears.

We suddenly feel anxious about becoming parents. Is this normal?

Yes. Having a baby is a time of great joy, but it's also normal to have feelings of uncertainty as the big day approaches. It can be useful to think of parenthood as rather like taking on a new job. It's exciting and different, but unknown, and we expect a bit of uncertainty as we learn the ropes. Talk to your partner about your new roles as parents. Listen to each other's concerns and don't be afraid to ask for help once the baby arrives.

I'm scared of the pain of giving birth. What can I do to prepare myself?

This is a completely normal feeling to have at this stage in your pregnancy, and you still have time to address your fears. If possible, talk to someone who knows you very well and whom you trust, about how you have dealt with pain in the past. When you compare labour with other painful experiences you may realize that you are stronger and more powerful than you thought. Research has shown that an important factor in improving the labour experience for women is to have good one-to-one support. Talk to your partner, your family, or your friends to find someone who will give you encouraging and positive support. You may be able to employ a birth supporter or doula. Doulas are trained and experienced in supporting labouring women. They can really help to reduce fear and anxiety and to promote good labour progress. Don't forget that there are effective methods of pain relief available to you in hospital (see pp 172–3). Talk to your midwife

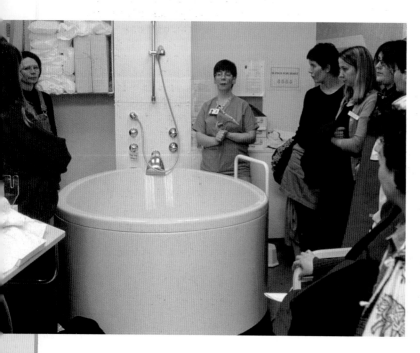

HOSPITAL TOUR *Face your fears about the birth by becoming informed. Familiarizing yourself with the hospital facilities, such as the birth pool, can help to prepare you for the big day.*

or doctor about these, and ask them to help you prepare a birth plan, so that your wishes are clear to everybody looking after you.

I think I'd be less anxious if I was booked in for a Caesarean. Is it an option?

It is important for you to understand that having a Caesarean will also involve pain, but after the birth, not before it. Although you will be given pain relief, you will have to recover from a major abdominal operation, with associated pain and weakness, for at least six weeks. It's also important to realize that you are more likely to develop complications, such as infection, it may take longer to conceive again and your baby is more likely to have breathing difficulties. Medical experts have differing views about opting for a Caesarean when there is no medical need. Some feel that it is not a good use of limited NHS funding, and that sometimes women who urgently need a Caesarean may not be able to have one quickly enough if the theatres are full of women having one by choice. Talk to your midwife about your fears of delivering naturally.

What if there's something wrong with my newborn baby?

Most parents-to-be have 'middle of the night' thoughts that there might be something wrong with their newborn baby, especially towards the end of the pregnancy. No one can be 100 per cent sure their baby is well until they hold him in their arms, but do remember that all the tests and scans you've had in pregnancy are designed to check that your baby is healthy. These days, if there is a problem with a baby, it is usually detected before birth. In the unlikely event that there is something wrong with your baby, be reassured that you will receive plenty of expert help and support from your doctors and midwives.

JUST FOR DAD

What you may be worried about now

Fears about the birth: Many fathers-to-be worry that they won't hold up during labour and delivery. You may worry about getting queasy, throwing up or even passing out in the presence of all those bodily fluids. Or you may simply find yourself dreading your partner's pain and worrying that you won't be a strong enough support person for her on the day. But while these are real and daunting emotional hurdles, most fathers navigate them just fine. Still, you should acknowledge your fears and anticipate your own limitations.

What you can do: Talking to other men who've been through the experience will give you some ideas about what you'll need to do to get through. You might also want to come up with some strategies for staying strong during your partner's labour and birth (see pp 150-151).

Plan to step out of the labour room when you need a breath of fresh air, for instance. Or talk to her about asking another relative or friend to offer back-up support. The two of you might even consider hiring a doula (see left) if you worry that you won't be in top form when the time comes.

Talk to your partner about developing a birth plan (see pp 166–7) so that you know her wishes, and define your role long before her contractions begin. And above all, read all you can about labour and delivery. If you and your partner haven't yet signed up for antenatal classes (see pp 132–3), do so right away – they are a great way to learn about labour and birth. That said, there's no way to prepare yourself for the profound joy of your baby's birth. You'll just have to feel it for yourself.

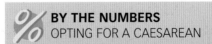

BY THE NUMBERS
OPTING FOR A CAESAREAN

Would you choose to have a Caesarean?

69% *No.*
22% *Yes.*
9% *Thinking about it.*

Source: Based on a BabyCentre.co.uk poll of 4,193 women.

How can we prepare for the birth and the first few weeks?

Your partner can play a very important role during labour and it helps if he has some idea of what to expect. Use the final weeks to talk about your expectations for the birth and read up on caring for your baby in the first few weeks.

Does my partner have to be the person with me during the birth?

Not necessarily. If your partner doesn't want to be at the birth, talk it through and decide what's right for both of you. If he isn't going to be there, you could consider enlisting the services of a close friend, your sister, your mother, or a paid birth companion called a doula (see p 148). For more information, contact the Doula UK (see p 227). If your birth companion is anyone other than your baby's father, tell your midwife.

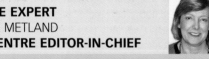

ASK THE EXPERT
DAPHNE METLAND
BABYCENTRE EDITOR-IN-CHIEF

Should my partner take full paternity leave or put his career first?

I would suggest that he does. He shouldn't feel he has to make a choice between that and his career. Society's underlying message is that men who make sacrifices and choose family over their career do it because they can't succeed at work. But we are at the beginning of an epic shift in cultural norms. More men are finding parenthood meaningful and that is raising the status of fathers. Some men are trading career advancement for time with their family because they value the fulfilment they find in fatherhood. The UK government's provision for parental leave (see p 117) is one way in which fathers are being increasingly recognized.

What can my partner do to prepare for the birth?

He should try to attend antenatal classes with you and talk through with you what you're hoping for at the birth. Write a birth plan together (see pp 166–7) so you can talk through things that matter to you. He may also find it useful to talk to other fathers who have been through the experience, although many men often only recall the wonder of seeing their baby born and not the labour process.

What is the role of a birth partner?

Primarily, to be there for you in any way you find comforting and useful. You can practise some of the ways your partner can help – massaging your lower back, for example. Do, however, keep an open mind, because you won't really know what you want until the day. It's important that you feel comfortable with each other – you may need to be very explicit about what you need! If medical intervention is suggested, your partner should ensure that you are aware of what is going on and seek clarification if necessary. But it's important that your partner doesn't cling to something you may have said before the event, not realizing that your views have now changed. He must be aware that you have the final word; although he might want to help you in making a decision, or in communicating that decision to the medical team.

I want my partner to be with me during the birth, but what if he finds it hard-going on the day?

Being a labour partner isn't for the faint-hearted: a first labour in particular may be many hours long. Providing emotional and physical support throughout is going to be exhausting, so your partner must look after himself, too. Talk beforehand about how and when he'll be able to take breaks, and make sure he remembers to take food and drink into hospital for himself. If the birth involves medical intervention, your partner may find it difficult to cope and may feel guilty about what is happening – make sure he, as well as you, talks this through afterwards with the midwife or obstetrician.

My partner is unsure what his role will be in the first few weeks. How can I reassure him?

This is a very common fear for men. The intense connection between a mother and a newborn – especially if the baby is being breastfed – can leave many men wondering whether the baby really needs them. Like many men, your partner might also doubt his ability to know how to care for the baby on a practical level, such as changing nappies and comforting him.

Reassure your partner that he will be an important person in your baby's life. From day one, your baby can be comforted and soothed by his dad. He can bond with him by holding, rocking and cooing at him. Taking over after feeds is a good opportunity, not least because it also gives you chance to recoup your energy. He can also help by lightening your workload around the house and giving you more relaxed time with your baby. You will be going through a really big learning curve and his emotional support is as important as his physical support.

Is there anything we can do to prepare for caring for our newborn?

Read parenting books together and discuss the issues that are raised, such as breastfeeding versus bottlefeeding and sleep safety. Besides offering helpful advice and food for thought, reading can give you something to do together in these final expectant months. Discuss your plans for how you will look after your baby and who you might ask to help in the first few weeks.

JUST FOR DAD

Preparing to be a dad

While your partner is busy counting tiny socks, you may start to wonder exactly what you should be doing, and begin to feel concerned about your role as a father. There are a million wonderful ways to be a great dad, and with a little patience and a lot of love, you will surely find your own. You don't need to earn lots of money, you don't need to own a football and you don't need to look the part. Just be true to yourself, and the rest will come naturally. Some men fear being like their own father, but your own father needn't be your role model for parenting. He is just one influence on what kind of dad you'll become. Look to others who have nurtured you over the years, including teachers, colleagues, friends, uncles, brothers and so on, and create your own identity as a father. Try to see fatherhood as a role you grow into.

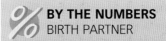

BY THE NUMBERS
BIRTH PARTNER

Who do you want to be with you during childbirth?

88% *Partner.*
6% *Relative.*
4% *No one besides medical staff.*
1% *Friend.*
1% *Doula.*

Source: Based on a BabyCentre.co.uk poll of 5,433 women.

Should we stop having sex now that I'm in the last trimester?

As long as your waters haven't broken and you don't have complications, there is no reason why you can't have sex right up to the time you go into labour. Although many women, understandably, find they aren't in the mood for lovemaking in the final weeks.

Is it safe to have sex in late pregnancy?

Yes, with a few exceptions. It's not safe, for instance, if you're bleeding or have placenta praevia (see p 37). You should also abstain from having sex after your waters break because then your baby is no longer protected against infection. It's also risky to have sex early in your third trimester if you're at risk of premature labour or if you have a weak cervix. In those cases an orgasm can stimulate dangerous contractions. But if you're having a healthy, normal pregnancy, there's no risk at all in having sex.

I'd still like sex, but it seems too much trouble. Should I make more effort?

Your feelings are understandable. Between the ever-bigger baby taking over your body, the various aches and indignities of late pregnancy, and your own preoccupation with the upcoming birth, sex may start to feel more like an acrobatic feat than an act of love. Plus, while those feisty baby kicks inflame your parenting excitement, they might not do much for your libido. If you do want to give it a go, just remember to keep a sense of humour. When the mood does strike, your body might seem uncooperative at best. Something has come between you and your partner – literally. Use your imagination and try different positions (see p 113) and be prepared to laugh a lot.

How can we stay close without sex?

Starting now, make the most of any sensual contact with your partner – massages, showering together, sleeping in the nude, mutual masturbation – even if it doesn't always end in intercourse. And even when you're not in the mood for sex, you can be affectionate with hugs, kisses and by saying "I love you". Finally, make sure your partner knows that it's

BabyCentre Buzz

"Massage is about as close to sexual excitement as it gets these days. We kiss, cuddle and snuggle all the time and, most importantly, talk about our feelings. My husband still misses sex, but we maintain intimacy. At this point, we're joking about how the first time we make love after the baby is born will be like 'the' first time' all over again." Louisa

"My husband's advice to other dads-to-be is this: instead of having sex, try patience, romance, massage, patience, understanding, patience!" Christine

"As I grow, my partner caresses my belly and looks at it like it's the most beautiful thing he's ever seen. I can think of nothing else that makes more of an impression on me. A lack of sex during pregnancy is something you get through just fine."hFiona

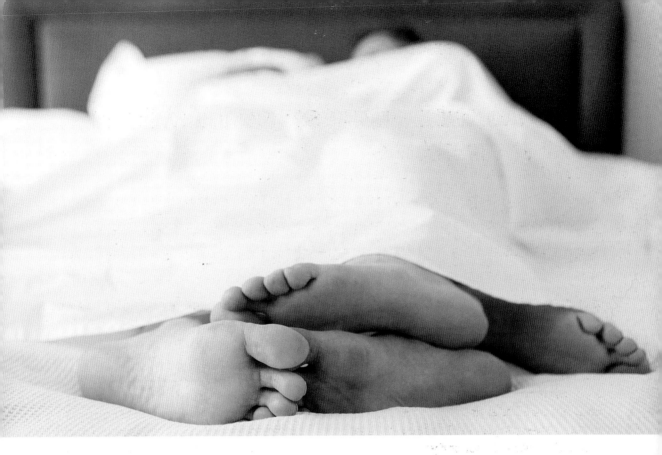

common for women to be less interested in sex late in pregnancy, and reassure him that this doesn't mean you love him any less.

I haven't wanted sex for months. Will my libido return once I've had my baby?

Your libido will return eventually, but don't expect it to be straight after your baby is born. During the early months with your newborn, fatigue, hormonal changes and generally adjusting to parenthood is likely to get in the way of sex. But give yourself time, and most importantly try not to let it become a problem between you and your partner.

Why is my vulva swollen?

This is due to varicose veins in your vulva. Like those in the legs, these painful swellings result from the weight of your growing uterus partially obstructing your blood flow, which increases pressure in the veins in the lower half of your body.

Avoid standing for long periods and try wearing waist-high support tights, going for walks, having warm baths, and lying down on your left side or with your legs raised (see p 137).

Why did I have cramps after I climaxed?

It is common to experience this problem during pregnancy. Your uterus contracts after orgasm even when you're not pregnant, but now you'll really be able to feel it. Do, however, let your midwife know if the contractions or pain continue for more than a few minutes and describe the pain if you can.

 QUICK TIP

If you are overdue, try having sex. It may trigger the release of a hormone that can increase the frequency of practice contractions. Semen also contains substances that soften the neck of the womb. If you think your waters may have broken, don't have sex as there is a risk of infection to your baby.

What should I be doing in the final weeks?

The last weeks of pregnancy can sometimes seem painfully long, but there is plenty you can be doing to prepare for your baby's arrival. It can be reassuring to know that you've finished work, your hospital bag is packed and you can focus on preparing yourself physically and emotionally for labour and birth.

JUST THE FACTS
WHAT TO PACK FOR LABOUR

The following items are useful during labour:

- *Your birth plan (see p 166).*
- *Dressing gown: useful if you end up pacing hospital corridors.*
- *Slippers and socks (believe it or not, your feet can get cold during labour) and an old nightdress or a T-shirt to wear in labour.*
- *Massage oil if you would like to be massaged.*
- *Lip balm because your lips may become dry during labour.*
- *Snacks and drinks for early labour, or some glucose tablets to keep you going.*
- *A watch with a second hand, or a stopwatch, to time contractions.*
- *Camera or camcorder, but check with the hospital that they are allowed.*
- *Relaxation materials, such as books and music.*
- *Pictures of someone or something you love.*
- *TENS pain relief machine (see p 170) if you are planning to use one.*
- *Water spray or hand-held fan to keep you cool.*
- *Clothes, toiletries, maternity pads and breast pads for after the birth.*
- *Car seat (the hospital may not let you leave without one if you're taking your baby home by car), nappies, clothes, blanket and muslin squares for your newborn.*

When should I pack my hospital bag and what can I take with me?

If you are planning a hospital birth, It's a good idea to have your bags packed (see left) by the time you are about 36 weeks pregnant in case your baby arrives early. Hospitals vary in their policies about what you are allowed to take with you when you have your baby. You may want to take a few items from home, such as your own cushions, to make the environment more personal. Check what the hospital provides and what you can bring yourself, but be aware that hospitals can be short on space.

Is it true that drinking raspberry leaf tea in the final weeks eases labour?

In a study carried out in Sydney, Australia, 192 first-time mums were given either a 1.2 g (½ oz) raspberry leaf tablet or a placebo twice a day from 32 weeks of pregnancy. The herb had no harmful effects, and those women who had taken raspberry leaf tablets were found to have a shorter second stage of labour and a lower rate of forceps delivery. However, far more research is needed to confirm these results. It's important not to use raspberry leaves until the last trimester because of their stimulating effect on the uterus. Start with one cup of tea a day (made with 1 tsp of raspberry leaf tea) or one tablet, and build up gradually to a maximum of four cups of tea or tablets daily.

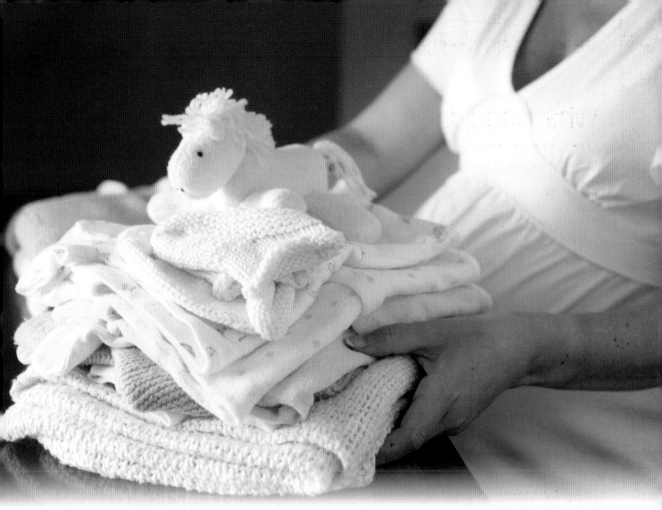

NESTING *It's believed that a spurt of nesting means that labour is just around the corner. If you're close to your due date you might be frantically organizing baby clothes and cleaning out cupboards – this is natural, but take time to rest. You'll need energy for the birth!*

What is perineal massage?

The perineum is the area of skin and muscle between the opening of your vagina and your anus. Perineal massage increases the elasticity of this area and reduces the risk of tearing or the need for an episiotomy (see p 182). To give the massage, put some vitamin E oil or pure vegetable oil on your fingers and thumbs and around your perineum. Place your thumbs inside your vagina and press downwards and sideways gently until you feel a slight tingling. Hold this stretch for about two minutes. Now gently massage the lower part of your vaginal canal for about three minutes, working the oil into the tissues.

How can I encourage my baby to get into the best position for birth?

You're more likely to have a straightforward birth if your baby has his spine facing towards the front of your bump. One way you can encourage your baby to take up what's known as the anterior position (see p 176) is by making sure your knees are always lower than your hips when sitting: use a cushion to lift up your bottom and bring your knees down. Kneeling on all fours for 10 minutes every day may also help.

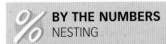

BY THE NUMBERS
NESTING

Did you notice the 'nesting instinct' in the weeks before you gave birth?

64% *Yes.*
36% *No.*

Source: Based on a BabyCentre. co.uk poll of 1,904 women.

What do I need to buy for my baby?

It's fun buying equipment and clothes in preparation for your baby's arrival, but the reality is that you need very little to care for a newborn in the first few weeks. So try not to be tempted by unnecessary items – just buy the essentials before your baby is born and hold off on buying any of the extras until later.

Is it okay to buy second-hand items?

The reality is that if it's available new, it's available second-hand. But not all baby items should be bought second-hand (see right). To get yourself started, try visiting a NCT (National Childbirth Trust) sale before your baby is born, to see the wide range of goods on sale. You'll probably find everything from baby cutlery to high-tech cloth nappies. And you'll find that many of the items will be virtually unused. Some second-hand items will cost a tenth of their original price or less.

As a rule of thumb, when buying second-hand items you should never pay more than a third of the full price. What you pay will depend in part on luck and determination and also where you choose to buy. Jumble sales and car boot sales are the bargain basement of the second-hand world, while online auctions can be quite expensive in comparison, but convenient. Certain items such as climbing frames can command up to half of their original price.

Which baby items shouldn't be bought second-hand?

You should not buy second-hand pushchairs or prams without the British Standard sticker BS7409, car seats, mattresses, baby bouncers and walkers, breast pumps, any mains-powered electrical items, hand-knitted toys, or any item of clothing with a drawstring around the neck.

In the case of second-hand toys, look for a CE Mark. Toys approved by the British Toy and Hobby Association will also carry the Lion Mark. You should also ensure the toy is suitable for your child's age group before buying it. Check the labels on nightwear to see if they say: 'Keep away from fire' and 'Low flammability to BS5722'. If not, they may not meet the latest safety standards.

Should I buy all newborn baby clothes or different sizes?

It's best to buy a mixture of sizes, not least because your baby may be born larger than you think. If you buy an outfit for a baby aged 3–6 months, bear in mind that it will be a different season by the time your baby wears it. Remember, also, that friends and family are likely to buy clothes as presents. Make sure everything you buy is machine-washable. Where possible, try to buy everything in 100 per cent cotton. Woolly or synthetic clothes can make a baby too hot and irritate his skin.

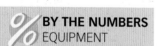

BY THE NUMBERS
EQUIPMENT

Did you go overboard when buying baby equipment?

54% *I bought just the right amount.*
32% *I bought far too much.*
7% *I bought too little.*
7% *I bought all the wrong things.*

Source: Based on a BabyCentre.co.uk poll of 370 women.

What is a travel system?

A travel system is a type of pushchair that is compatible with a rear-facing car seat and usually a carrycot. The car seat and carrycot can both click in and out of the pushchair, which can be very handy when you have a sleeping baby that you don't want to wake up. Although travel systems may seem expensive, they are economical because you get a pushchair and separate car seat. The carrycot can be used as an alternative to a Moses basket for your baby to sleep in.

What size car seat should I buy?

Car seat sizes can seem confusing, as there are several different systems used to categorize them. Some people talk about Group 0 and 0+ car seats, others refer to Stage 1 or 2. The retail trade now refers to seats by Groups, to try and avoid confusion. It's simpler if you think in terms of choosing the right seat for your baby's weight using the following guide: from birth to 10 kg (22 lb) (newborn to nine months) choose group 0; from birth to 13 kg (27 lb) (newborn to 15–18 months) choose group 0+; for 9 kg–18 kg (20–40 lb) (9 months–4 years) choose group 1.

Should I buy a sling to carry my baby?

Yes, slings and carriers have many advantages. They let you keep your baby close to you but still have your hands free for other activities. Many parents find that running errands and even doing housework is easier when their baby is carried along. If you have two children, slings and carriers can save you the cost of buying a double pushchair. Your young baby can be supported in a baby carrier while the eldest child is in a pushchair. Small babies often like the feel of being carried about in a sling or carrier and will often happily go to sleep in them.

JUST THE FACTS
WHAT YOU NEED TO BUY

These are the essential items you need to buy before your baby is born.

- **Nappies** *Newborns need their nappies changed as often as 10–12 times a day so buy enough for at least the first few days. If you are planning to use reusable nappies, it's a good idea to have at least one pack of disposables too.*

- **Baby wipes or cotton wool** *Needed for nappy changing.*

- **Changing mat** *or a changing unit.*

- **All-in-one sleepsuits** *Seven sleepsuits will be very handy. Small babies don't need to wear anything else, apart from a vest in winter months, or a cardigan if it is very cold.*

- **Baby vests/body suits** *At least three or four vests with envelope necks and poppers underneath, also known as body suits, are essential. These can be worn under a sleepsuit or, when the weather is very hot, a baby vest may be all your baby needs to wear.*

- **One or two blankets** *to keep your baby warm.*

- **One or two cardigans** *as an extra layer.*

- **All-in-one warm suit** *Essential if your baby is born in winter.*

- **Moses basket, cot or crib** *plus a new mattress that fits properly.*

- **Cot sheets and cellular blankets** *or a bottom sheet and a baby sleeping bag.*

- **Baby bath** *(or washing-up bowl), or a newborn bath support. Plus a couple of small towels and some mild baby bath.*

- **Rear-facing car seat** *if your baby will be travelling home from hospital by car.*

- **Pram, pushchair or buggy** *Buy one with a lie-flat position that is suitable for newborns.*

- **Nursing bras and breast pads** *for breast-feeding, or bottles, teats, bottle brushes and a sterilizing method, if you plan to bottlefeed.*

How should I deal with unwanted advice?

There's nothing quite like a baby to generate excitement and following swiftly behind will come the advice. Baby names, birth plans, breastfeeding – you name it and someone will have an opinion on it. Listen as patiently as you can, but always remember your first responsibility is to yourself, your partner and your new baby.

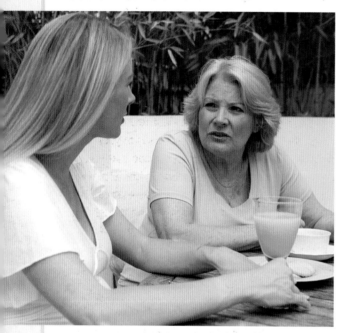

BEING TRUE TO YOURSELF As advice pours in, try to keep a respectful attitude and an open mind, but stay in touch with your own instincts. Remember that times have changed since your parents had their children and you'll know what's best for yours.

How can I make sure I involve my mum in my pregnancy, but also keep a healthy distance between us?

The attentions of a super-keen granny-to-be can be a little suffocating when you're expecting, and you may find that you need to put a few boundaries in place. Take the initiative and decide how much time you feel comfortable spending with your mother, how often you would like to chat to her on the telephone, and so on. It's also important to think about how you see your mum fitting into your life once your baby has arrived.

Make it plain that you are interested in her life outside the family, and make a point of talking about topics other than babies. Remind yourself that your mother will have valuable experience that could be really helpful to you as a new mum. Asking her advice sometimes can help you grow closer in a new, positive way.

My dad disapproves because we're not planning to marry now that I'm pregnant. How should I handle this?

To your dad, marriage probably means safety and security for you and your family, so he'd understandably want this for you. Perhaps you and your partner never intend to get married and, eventually, your dad will grow used to the idea. However, if it's important for you to have his understanding and support now, it may help to explain why you've decided not to marry. So that this doesn't become an issue throughout your pregnancy, you and your partner will need to talk to your dad in an adult way about the decision you've taken, explaining your reasons calmly and clearly. If you're worried about your emotions overwhelming you when you speak to him, try practising what you'll say out loud beforehand.

My mother-in-law has become overbearing now she knows she's going to be a grandmother. What can I do?

This problem gives you and your partner a good opportunity to work together. This is not just your responsibility but your partner's, too; it's his mother after all. Talk with him about the way it makes you feel. Ask him how he can help you to deal with it.

You don't want to alienate your mother-in-law; after all she means no harm. It's also great to have offers of help and support once the baby is born, as long as they are on your terms. Your partner should explain to his mother that it's good to know she's there and that you'll ask for help when you need it.

How can I stop people telling me their negative birth stories?

The birth process is a very powerful and memorable one for most women. As you've discovered, people love to have an opportunity to tell you about their own experiences, which may not always be positive. If you find a friend launching into what you know is going to be a draining story for you, interrupt her before she really gets going. If you are going to antenatal classes, explain that you are already learning all the latest techniques and ideas on birth, which you find reassuring and helpful. Tell people that you would like to talk with them about their birth experiences, but would prefer to do this when you've got your own delivery story to add to theirs.

People are disapproving when I tell them I want a home birth. What can I do?

Equipping yourself with evidence about the safety of home birth (see pp 168–9) is probably the best way of dealing with this – you will counteract other people's negativity as well as reassuring yourself. Take every opportunity to ask your midwife and other women who have had home deliveries as many questions as you can about what it involves. Getting your partner's support and understanding will help you to deal with negative comments in a confident and assertive way. It may also be a good idea to mention to people who are critical that your doctor and midwife are happy with your decision to give birth to your baby at home.

How can I help my mum learn to respect my decision to go back to work?

This is about your mum accepting you as an adult who can make well-informed decisions about the way you want to run your life. It's also about her accepting that ideas about parenting, work and lifestyle have changed over the last few decades.

Explaining your thoughts and ideas to your mum in a calm way will help her to see that you are a responsible adult. Try talking to her with your partner there, too, so that she can see that you both agree on this decision. By behaving in a thoughtful, informed, caring and reasonable way, you will probably earn your mum's respect.

BabyCentre Buzz

"*My mum would prefer it if I stopped working now that I'm pregnant and didn't return to work after the baby is born. But we talked it through and I think she understands my decision now.*" Katie

"*When people gave me advice, I just tried to be positive as I knew they meant well. As long as you are positive about your choices, people will respect them.*" Zahara

"*My in-laws are generous to a fault but also very controlling. They started buying baby items – even nursery furniture! – soon after we'd announced the pregnancy. My husband had a quiet word...*" Lynne

Can I still go out and about?

There should be no reason why you can't go out and about in the final weeks of pregnancy. It can help to relieve the boredom as you await your baby's arrival and a little gentle exercise may be beneficial. However, you might not want to stray too far from home, just in case!

Is it wise to travel in the last few weeks?

It depends on your circumstances, but you will probably find you don't want to go very far. Complaints such as back pain, swelling and general fatigue can make travelling more punishing than pleasurable. You might also get anxious if you're far away from home – most women prefer to be near to home or their hospital. If you're planning to take a long trip, check with your midwife first. If you're just going out locally try to get lifts whenever you can. Driving can be tiring and uncomfortable in the later stages of pregnancy.

What should I take with me when I'm out and about in the final weeks?

Carry your personal maternity record (see p 84), which should include your due date, risk factors, blood type, a list of medications you're taking and any that you're allergic to. Keep this with you at all times in the last few weeks. Prepare a complete list of names and phone numbers to contact in case of an emergency and keep it in your bag.

How can I stay comfortable while travelling by car?

Sitting anywhere for long periods of time can make your feet and ankles swell and your legs cramp. Keep your blood circulating by taking a break from

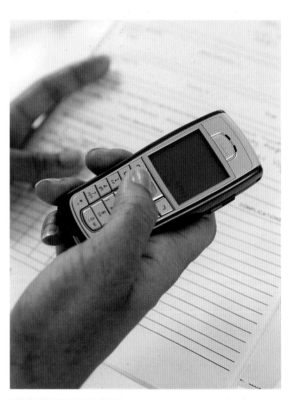

EMERGENCY CONTACTS *Put any emergency contact details, such as your midwife's phone number, into your mobile phone or keep a list of them in your bag. Make sure you keep your personal maternity record (see p 84) with you wherever you go.*

driving at least every 90 minutes. (You may need to stop that often for toilet breaks anyway.) Pull over at a rest area to walk around and do some simple stretches. If you're a passenger, keep your seat reclined to a comfortable position (with your seat

BabyCentre Buzz

"We went out locally in the final weeks of my pregnancy. It was relaxing, but without the hassle of too much planning or the anxiety of being away." June

"I tended to stay home a lot towards the end of my pregnancy. When I was 38 weeks pregnant, I had a spa day at my house and invited friends over for an afternoon of manicures and facials." Susan

"My husband and I had a weekend 'away' a week before the baby was due, but were only in the local hotel. We used their wonderful swimming pool and had a lovely dinner in the hotel restaurant." Natalie

belt on), and try these simple exercises: extend your leg, heel first, and gently flex your foot to stretch your calf muscles. Then rotate your ankles clockwise and anticlockwise and wiggle your toes.

Will wearing a seat belt harm my unborn baby in any way?

Not if you wear your seat belt correctly. Make sure the lap belt is secured below your bump and across your hips. It should lie snugly over your pelvis. The shoulder belt should fit snugly over your bump and between your breasts. If it cuts across your neck, try repositioning your seat so the belt fits better. Never wear the belt across your belly – during a crash, the sudden jolt could damage the placenta and put your baby at risk.

What should I do if I have contractions away from home?

First of all, don't panic. Remember that labour usually takes many hours. Call your midwife or the hospital and you will be given advice on what to do

depending on your stage of pregnancy, the rate of your contractions and where you are. If you're in the car, don't drive.

I'm already desperate for a holiday. How soon after giving birth can my baby and I safely take a trip?

For most new mothers who have had few, if any, complications and are recuperating well, travelling (as long as it isn't too strenuous) one to two weeks after a vaginal delivery and three to four weeks after a Caesarean is fine. But it's also important during this time to listen carefully to the signals your body is sending.

Remember that recovery from childbirth takes time, rest and assistance. Even if you planned a trip while you were pregnant, don't go on it if you're not feeling up to it once the baby is born. Travel can be stressful, and if you've taken a long flight, jet lag can compound the fatigue you're already experiencing. The first few weeks after delivery can be emotionally difficult as well (see pp 206–7). Breastfeeding (see pp 198–9), especially for first-time mums, can sometimes take time to get established.

If you've got lots of stitches they may feel uncomfortable for some time, and can be made worse by vigorous exercise. Regardless of your mode of travel, take it as easy as possible. If your pregnancy was complicated, always carry a copy of your medical records with you.

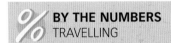

% BY THE NUMBERS
TRAVELLING

What's the hardest part of travelling during pregnancy?

37% *Needing the toilet.*
22% *Fatigue.*
13% *Worries about miscarriage.*
10% *Swollen feet.*
10% *Worries about labour.*
8% *It's no harder than before pregnancy.*

Source: Based on a BabyCentre.co.uk poll of 682 women.

How will our baby fit into our family?

The arrival of a new baby is a wonderful event, which is likely to enhance your life and the lives of your immediate family in many ways. However, be aware that a newborn will, inevitably, change the dynamics of family life. It's especially important to prepare any existing children for your baby's arrival.

How can we help our three-year-old bond with our new baby?

The first meeting is often seen as a crucial test of the sibling relationship, but most people believe it has little bearing in the long term. All the same, you want to get it right. Try to make sure your new baby is in his cot when your toddler comes in, so your arms are open and ready for a cuddle, as always. If you're in hospital, have some treats lined up to give your toddler when she visits to ease her time at home without you. Make your toddler aware from the very start that the baby is interested in her, is watching her and loves her. Involve your toddler in games with your baby, and always tell her how much you value her assistance at bathtime or with tasks such as fetching a nappy.

Should I potty train my toddler before the baby arrives?

Although it's the ideal wish for many parents that their toddler is out of nappies before the next baby comes, potty training should start at an appropriate time for your particular child. This is because its success is dependent on nerve-path maturity, and your toddler having the physical and cognitive skills to manage. Between two and two-and-a-half years is the time when many children seem to be aware of being wet and dirty and you have a better chance of succeeding in training them. Boys are usually later at achieving this than girls.

Luckily, that crucial age of opportunity often corresponds to the average age gap between siblings. However, if possible, try not to initiate anything immediately before a major life event, such as the arrival of a baby. If you force the issue and try potty training too early, you may come up against a strong-willed individual who refuses to comply. This causes tension all round and the key to successful potty training is to be as relaxed as possible. Be aware that setbacks can

ASK THE EXPERT
ANNA MCGRAIL
BABYCENTRE EXECUTIVE EDITOR

We have children from previous relationships. How can we help them accept our new baby?

For many children living in blended families, the arrival of a new baby equals the realization that their parents will never get back together. It can cause disruption and upset to children who have already gone through bereavement or the break-up of their parents' relationship. But it can and often does work – your older children might just need time to adapt. A large age gap between your existing children and the new baby is not necessarily a disadvantage. Many older siblings may be pleased to help with babycare, but don't take advantage of their good nature and expect them to babysit all the time, or to change lots of nappies. A new baby can bring happiness, but it may take time and you should expect moments of jealousy.

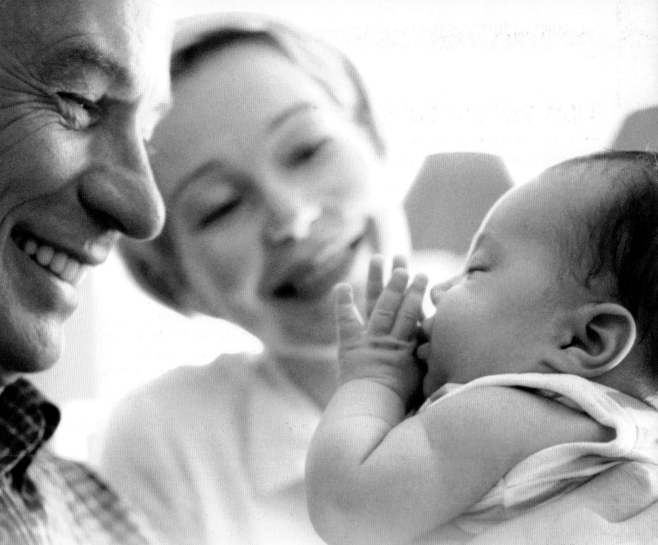

GRANDPARENTS AS CARERS Asking your own parents to be your baby's carers can be the perfect and cheapest arrangement. You'll be certain that your baby is getting lots of love and attention, but to avoid conflict make sure you are in agreement about childcare issues.

be common with the arrival of a second baby, with approximately half of all potty-trained toddlers wetting themselves again. This is a perfectly normal response to change and is usually short-lived.

Is it unwise to ask my mother to look after the baby when I return to work?

No, not necessarily. Care by a relative has been around as long as mothers have needed help taking care of their babies – basically, since time began. And it's still a popular solution for many parents today. This arrangement has its pluses – you can be fairly sure that your mother will have your child's best interests at heart, for instance. But there are minuses, too: it may be difficult giving your own mother pointers on how to care for her grandchild. The arrangement works best for people who have good relationships with relatives who, in turn, are flexible and are willing and able to help.

You also have to be prepared to establish a businesslike relationship with your mother. If that makes you uncomfortable, then this arrangement may not work for you. If your mother is willing and able to take care of your child and she shares your values and views on childrearing, consider yourself lucky. As long as you and your mother start out with a healthy relationship and maintain it, this inexpensive childcare option is likely to provide your child with more love and security than any other.

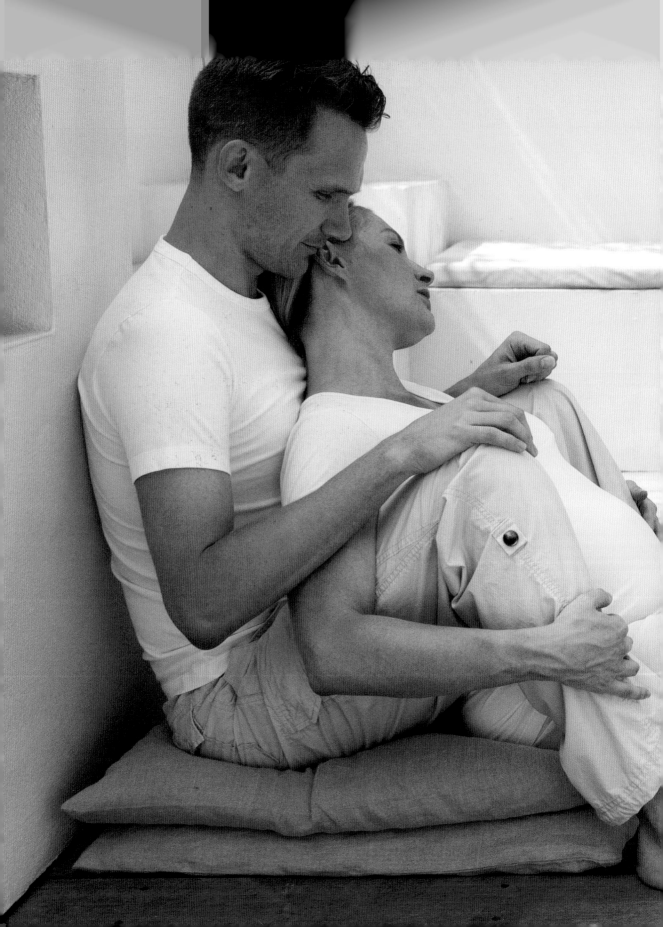

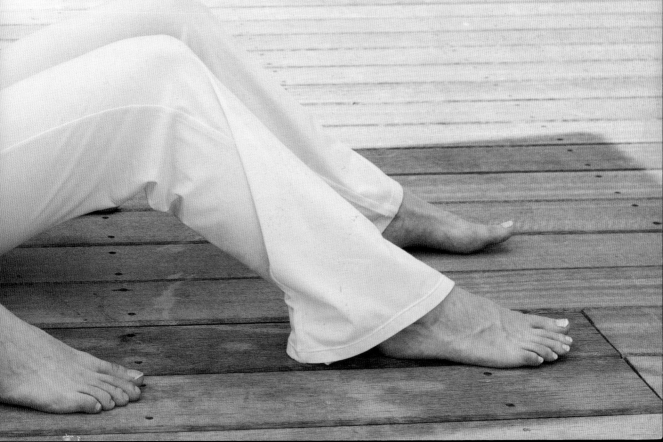

Labour and birth

Your entire pregnancy and all of your preparations have led to
this moment, and your baby will soon be in your arms. Being informed
about what might happen during labour and birth can give you more
confidence throughout the experience, but try to keep an open mind.

How can I prepare for the birth?

Whether you're planning a home or hospital birth, it's natural to have strong feelings about how your labour is managed. By writing a birth plan, you can make your wishes known about issues such as pain relief. Work with your midwife as you prepare for the birth; she is there to help and advise.

What is a birth plan?

A birth plan is a way of communicating with the midwives and doctors who care for you in labour. It is a record of what you would like to happen during your labour and after the birth. It's not written in tablets of stone because the best birth plans acknowledge that things may not go according to plan. Discussing the content with your midwife will give you the chance to ask questions and find out

more information. During labour she may need to recommend a course of action different from that you had originally hoped for, but which is in the best interests of your baby. Make sure your birth partner is aware of your wishes, too.

What are my options when it comes to the birth itself?

If you have a choice of where to have your baby, you can visit local hospitals and birth centres to find out about their procedures and decide which suits you best. Wherever you give birth, you can choose to have gas and air, or an injection for pain relief (see pp 172–3) if you need it, or nothing at all. Not every hospital has a birthing pool or 24-hour availability of epidurals so check this first if you think you might like either of these.

If your labour is slow, your midwife or doctor may recommend speeding it up (see pp 188–9), but you do not have to agree. You can choose your position for giving birth, though if you have an epidural (see pp 174–5) the positions are more limited as your legs will feel numb. Your baby's heartbeat may be monitored electronically (see pp 180–1) and the reasons for this should be explained. You can choose to have your baby delivered straight on to your tummy, and your partner may like to cut the umbilical cord. You can choose to allow the placenta to come away on its own or have an injection (see pp 184–5).

ASK THE EXPERT
CHRISSIE HAMMONDS
MIDWIFE SONOGRAPHER

What is a birth centre and how does it differ from a hospital?

Birth centres are small maternity units that are staffed and, in most cases, run by midwives. Birth centres may also be known as 'midwife-led units', 'birthing centres', 'maternity homes or hospitals' or 'GP units'. Most birth centres are independent, but lots of hospitals are opening midwife-led centres alongside conventional maternity units. Birth centres are a halfway house between home and hospital, offering a comfortable, low-tech environment where birth is treated as a 'normal' rather than a medical process. However, they are well equipped and staffed with highly skilled midwives. Birth centres can offer facilities that may not be available in hospital, such as family accommodation, birth pools, complementary therapies and low-tech birthing rooms. You are more likely to have one-to-one care from a midwife in a birth centre.

Is a water birth an option in hospital?

If you would like to labour and/or give birth to your baby in water, talk to your midwife about it at one of your antenatal appointments. She will be able to tell you if the hospital that you are booked into for the birth has a pool available and in use. About half of all hospitals have facilities for women to labour or give birth in water, but some may be more encouraging about their use than others. Maternity units should ensure that their midwives are trained to be competent, confident and skilled in assisting women who choose to labour or deliver in water.

How long will I have to stay in hospital?

If you have a normal birth and no complications, it's likely that you will be ready to go home the day after your baby is born or even on the same day. If you have a Caesarean (see pp 192–3), you may need to stay in hospital for 3–7 days. If you or your baby has any medical problems, you will have to stay in hospital longer. Some new mothers love being looked after and feel safe in hospital; others can't wait to get home.

BEING INFORMED *Hospital delivery rooms are equipped to medically manage the birth of your baby if necessary, but you do have a say. Ask your midwife about the different equipment and procedures that are used in your particular hospital.*

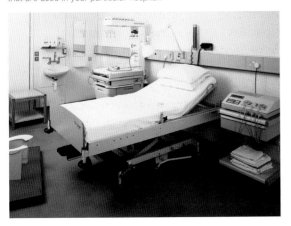

JUST THE FACTS
YOUR BIRTH PLAN

Consider the following in your birth plan:

- **Birth companion** *Write down who you want to be with you in labour. Do you want this person to stay with you all the time?*

- **Positions for labour and birth** *Mention which positions you would like to use and how active you would like to be.*

- **Pain relief** *State what methods you want to use, if any, and in what order (see pp 172–3).*

- **Birth pool** *If your hospital or midwife-led unit has a birth pool, or if you are hiring one to use at home, write down whether you want to use it for pain relief and/or to give birth in.*

- **Monitoring** *State how you want your baby to be monitored during labour. If your labour is progressing normally, the midwife will listen to your baby's heartbeat at regular intervals to check for any changes in the heart rate. She may suggest electronic monitoring (see pp 180–1), perhaps after you have pain relief, or if your baby is showing signs of distress.*

- **Assisted delivery** *You might want to express a preference for forceps or ventouse (see pp 190–1) if you need some help to deliver your baby. Bear in mind that, in the end, the position of your baby may dictate the method used.*

- **Delivery of the placenta** *You can have an injection to speed up the delivery of the placenta, or you might prefer to have a natural third stage without drugs (see pp 184–5).*

- **Feeding your baby** *Be clear about whether you want to breastfeed (see pp 198–9) or bottlefeed (see pp 200–1). If you want to breastfeed and don't want your baby to have bottles, say so.*

- **Special needs** *If you have particular religious needs, make sure that you include these. For example, it might be important for you to have certain rituals carried out when your baby is born, or you might require a special diet.*

What can I expect from a home birth?

Research shows that a planned home birth is just as safe as a hospital birth, but you may be advised against it if your pregnancy is considered to be high-risk. The likelihood of you needing medical intervention is reduced by home birth, but you will be transferred to hospital if your midwife thinks it is necessary.

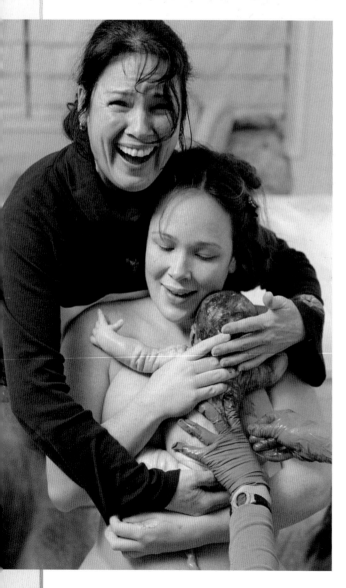

Can I choose to have a home birth?

According to government guidelines, women should be supported in their childbirth choices and, though the majority of women still have their babies in hospital, many more are choosing to have a home birth. Most midwives and doctors are supportive of women's wishes, but you may come up against a doctor or a midwife who feels strongly that you should book for a hospital birth. Of course, they may have a very good reason. If you have a history of postnatal haemorrhage or are expecting twins, for example, you would probably be wise to have a hospital birth, as there may be complications. On the other hand, if you are advised by a midwife or doctor to go into hospital simply because you're having your first baby, ask them why. There's no evidence that you're putting yourself or your baby at greater risk by opting for a home birth.

How do I organize a home birth?

Speak to your doctor or midwife after your pregnancy has been confirmed. If your doctor isn't keen on a home birth, don't worry as you don't need his or her consent. Ask to be referred to a community midwife or doctor who will provide full

HOME COMFORTS *Having your baby at home, where the surroundings are familiar and comfortable, can be a calmer, more personal and less clinical experience. It also gives you the opportunity to have other family members or friends present.*

maternity services. Or write to the manager of your local community midwifery services – get her name and address from your local maternity unit. She will contact you to make the arrangements. Another option is to pay an independent midwife, who can carry out your antenatal care, attend the birth of your baby at home if all goes to plan and provide postnatal care, but this can be costly.

What if I change my mind about having a home birth?

Your doctors and midwives should provide a flexible system of care so that you have plenty of time to decide where you are going to give birth, and alter that decision close to your due date if you so wish. Opting for a home birth allows you the greatest possible flexibility, as you can decide to transfer to hospital right up to the delivery itself, whereas swapping from a hospital to a home birth may not be possible due to practical considerations.

What happens if I need to have hospital treatment during labour?

Your midwife will talk to you and your partner about why she believes a transfer to hospital would be a good idea and will then call an ambulance. This sounds very dramatic, but in fact you're far more likely to need to transfer to hospital because your labour has slowed down than because there's a real emergency. At the hospital, the midwife who has been at your home will still look after you, unless for any reason she can't carry on, in which case another midwife will take over your care.

What equipment do I need?

Very little – a few weeks before your due date, your midwife will bring round a birth pack containing all the bits and pieces she needs. All you may be

BabyCentre Buzz

"I've decided to try a home birth with my first baby and am currently 18 weeks pregnant. I expected huge hostility from my midwives but they seemed more excited than dismayed at the prospect." Aisha

"Do your research and be assertive. However, don't be too inflexible – sometimes there are good reasons why hospital is a safer option." Stephanie

"Having a home birth made having my second child a much easier and hassle-free experience. It was great giving birth and being able to eat pizza and watch TV at the same time!" Angela

asked to provide is an angle-poise lamp, which can be used to check your perineum (the area between the vagina and anus) after the delivery, and perhaps a portable heater. If you are planning a water birth you will need to arrange for a birth pool to be delivered to your house some weeks before your due date. Your midwife or your local National Childbirth Trust branch (see p 228) will be able to tell you where you can hire one. Your partner should start filling the pool as soon as your labour begins. Don't wait until you need to use it!

What happens after the birth?

Once your baby is born and the placenta is safely delivered (see pp 184–5), the midwives will probably leave you and your partner alone with your baby for a while. They'll then check and weigh your baby, help you with your first breastfeed and clear up any mess. Your midwife or another community midwife will then visit you every day for a few days to check your baby and see how you're progressing. Your doctor will also usually call on the first day and carry out a complete check on your baby.

How can I ease the pain naturally?

If you want to remain in control during labour and have minimal medical intervention, it's worth familiarizing yourself with a few ways in which you can manage the pain of contractions. Breathing, movement, massage and labouring in water can all help you to relax and beat labour pain naturally.

Does massage during labour really help?

Yes. Massage stimulates the body to release endorphins, which are natural pain-killing and mood-lifting substances. Endorphins are responsible for the 'high' you feel after vigorous exercise, or a good laugh with friends. Research has shown that women who are massaged during labour are less anxious and experience less pain as well as having shorter labours and less postnatal depression (see pp 208–9) than women who are not massaged. However, some women simply cannot bear to be touched when they are having contractions. Birth companions need to be aware of these different reactions and respond accordingly.

Can certain labour positions help to ease the pain?

Research, though limited, has shown that women who remain mobile during labour have shorter labours and fewer drugs for pain relief than those who take to their bed. However, when the contractions are very strong, you will probably find that you don't want to move around a great deal. You'll need all your strength simply to cope with each contraction as it comes along. Most women naturally find the position that suits them best. Just keep rocking, leaning forwards during contractions and straightening up in between.

Does being in water during labour help?

Yes, being in water during labour can make contractions more bearable, just as having a bath can help to ease backache. Two important studies have found that using a birth pool significantly reduces women's use of pain-relieving drugs in labour. Women expecting their first babies and who

ASK THE EXPERT
LESLEY PAGE
PROFESSOR OF MIDWIFERY

What is a TENS machine and how does it help to relieve pain during labour?

TENS stands for Transcutaneous Electrical Nerve Stimulation. A TENS machine consists of a small box with a clip on the back so you can attach it to your clothes. The machine gives out little pulses of electrical energy through four wires connected to sticky pads. Two pads are placed on either side of your spine at about bra-strap level and two at about the level of the dimples in your bottom. The pads are covered in a gel to help the electrical pulses pass through your skin more easily. The TENS machine has dials that you can adjust to control the frequency and strength of the pulses. There's also a boost button for you to hold and press when you want maximum output. TENS works best at the beginning of labour because it takes about an hour for your body to respond to the electrical impulses by releasing endorphins. It's advisable to hire a TENS machine and use it before you go into hospital – very few hospitals provide them.

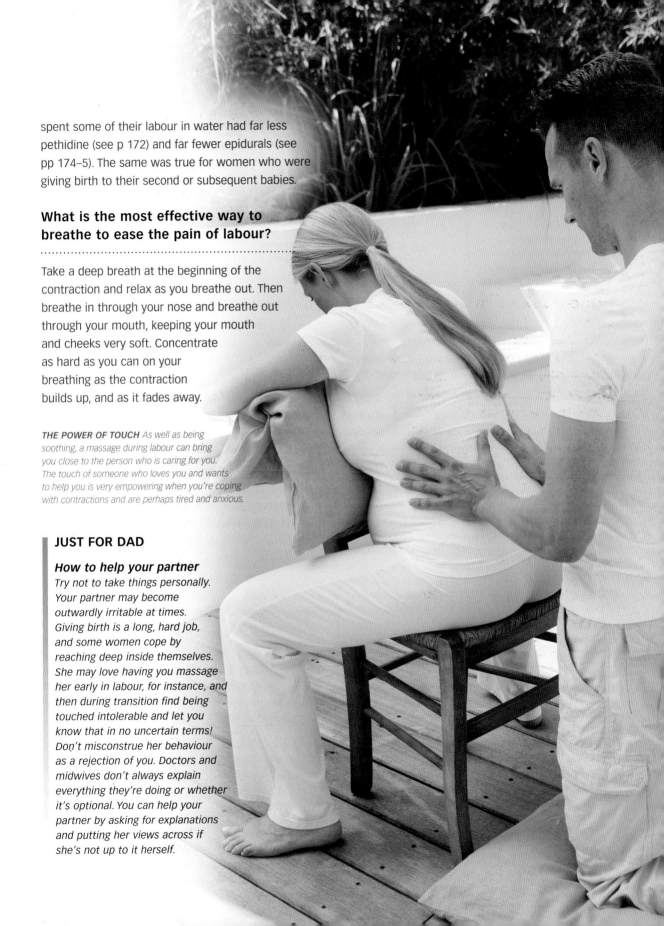

spent some of their labour in water had far less pethidine (see p 172) and far fewer epidurals (see pp 174–5). The same was true for women who were giving birth to their second or subsequent babies.

What is the most effective way to breathe to ease the pain of labour?

Take a deep breath at the beginning of the contraction and relax as you breathe out. Then breathe in through your nose and breathe out through your mouth, keeping your mouth and cheeks very soft. Concentrate as hard as you can on your breathing as the contraction builds up, and as it fades away.

THE POWER OF TOUCH As well as being soothing, a massage during labour can bring you close to the person who is caring for you. The touch of someone who loves you and wants to help you is very empowering when you're coping with contractions and are perhaps tired and anxious.

JUST FOR DAD

How to help your partner
Try not to take things personally. Your partner may become outwardly irritable at times. Giving birth is a long, hard job, and some women cope by reaching deep inside themselves. She may love having you massage her early in labour, for instance, and then during transition find being touched intolerable and let you know that in no uncertain terms! Don't misconstrue her behaviour as a rejection of you. Doctors and midwives don't always explain everything they're doing or whether it's optional. You can help your partner by asking for explanations and putting her views across if she's not up to it herself.

What are my pain-relief options?

Medical pain relief during labour, such as gas and air or an epidural will be available to you during labour. Nobody knows exactly how labour will feel for them – some women find it is bearable with little or no pain relief, although many need help at some point. It's best to be informed about the advantages and disadvantages of each method.

What is an epidural?

An epidural is an injection into the small of your back that numbs the lower part of your abdomen so that you can't feel the pain of the contractions. It usually numbs the feet and legs too. The curved, hollow needle goes between the vertebrae of your spine, and into the space around your spinal cord. A fine tube is passed through the needle and then the needle is removed. The tube is taped up your back and over your shoulder. The anaesthetist injects a local anaesthetic into the tube. (See pp 174–5 for more on epidurals.)

What is pethidine and how is it given?

Pethidine is an analgesic (a painkiller) but also an anti-spasmodic, which is a drug that helps you relax. It works in a similar way to morphine – in fact, it is a synthetic version of morphine. Your midwife can both prescribe and administer injections of pethidine for pain relief without consulting a doctor first. Pethidine can be given intravenously and is often combined with another drug – an anti-emetic – to control sickness.

A fine tube is inserted into a vein in your arm and the other end of the tube is attached to a pump that you can operate to give yourself small amounts of pethidine. This is called Patient Controlled Analgesia or PCA, but it's not available everywhere. Pethidine is given during the first stage of labour when your cervix is opening up from being tightly closed to 10 cm dilated; that is, before you start pushing. You can't have pethidine if your midwife thinks you're close to giving birth because it can affect your baby. Although pethidine can help you relax, the downside is that it can make you very sleepy or dizzy and causes some women to vomit, and it may slow labour down. Pethidine does cross the placenta and may affect your baby's breathing. Your baby may need to have an injection

ASK THE EXPERT
LESLEY PAGE
PROFESSOR OF MIDWIFERY

What is a spinal injection and why might I need one during labour?

This is an injection of local anaesthetic into the small of your back, which numbs the nerves supplying your uterus and cervix so that you can't feel contractions. Spinals are usually given in the second stage of labour to provide pain relief quickly if you are going to have a forceps or ventouse birth (see pp 190–1) and you haven't got an epidural in place. They are sometimes used in the first stage in conjunction with an epidural – this technique gives pain relief faster and is more popular than an epidural alone. On the upside, a spinal provides very effective and rapid pain relief in a single injection and, unlike an epidural, there is no tube left in your back. On the downside, it limits your mobility because you won't be able to feel your legs, it is short acting and can't be topped up. It may make you feel shivery, itchy or sick, and cause difficulties passing urine.

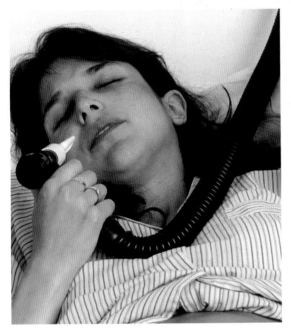

EASING THE PAIN *Entonox, also known as 'gas and air', is the mildest form of medical pain relief and the one many women start with in the early stages of labour. It will not prevent the use of other methods of pain relief if you feel you need something stronger.*

as soon as she is born to reverse the effects of the pethidine in her system. It can make the baby sleepy for a few days and not interested in feeding.

What is Entonox and how do I use it during labour?

Entonox, often called 'gas and air', is a colourless and odourless gas made up of 50 per cent oxygen and 50 per cent nitrous oxide (an analgesic). The vast majority of maternity hospitals pump Entonox to all of their delivery rooms from a central supply, so it's always available when you want it. If you are offered a face mask, place it over your face and inhale through your nose. If you are given a mouthpiece simply put it between your lips or teeth and breathe deeply and evenly. Continue to breathe deeply until you start to feel a little light-headed. Your hand will then drop away from your face and

you will stop breathing in the Entonox. Within a few seconds, you will feel perfectly normal again. Start breathing the Entonox the very second you feel a contraction beginning. It takes at least 20 seconds for the gas to build up in your bloodstream to a sufficient level to give you some pain relief, and 45–50 seconds before it reaches its greatest effectiveness.

The advantages of Entonox are that it's easy to use, is controlled by you and doesn't stay in your system (it also contains oxygen, which is good for your baby). On the downside it is only a mild painkiller, may make you feel sick and make your mouth feel dry.

Can I use pain relief if I'm in a birth pool?

Yes, but the methods of pain relief that can be used in a birth pool are more restricted. It's safe to use gas and air because the gas is not strong enough to make you feel out of control, and you are at no risk of slipping under the water because of its effects. Gas and air is usually brought to the pool room in a cylinder. If you're having your baby at home, your midwife will bring a cylinder with her when you go into labour. You can't have pethidine (see left) if you're in a pool because it will make you drowsy or have an epidural (see left and pp 174–5) because it will limit your mobility. A TENS machine (see p 170) can't be used because it is electrical and therefore is not compatible with water. However, the calming effect of the water should help you to manage the pain naturally.

QUICK TIP

If you're offered 'gas and air' through a rubber face mask, and the smell of rubber makes you feel queasy, ask for a plastic mouthpiece. It's easy to swap the mask for a mouthpiece. Sip water in between contractions to keep your mouth moist.

Having an epidural

Many women choose to have an epidural because it provides effective pain relief during labour. You may already know that you want one or you may not decide until you're actually having the contractions. Either way, it's advisable to be aware of both the advantages and disadvantages.

How an epidural works

An epidural contains the same anaesthetic that is used to numb the mouth before a tooth is extracted. It works by deadening the nerves that carry pain signals from your uterus and cervix so that you can't feel the contractions. Epidurals are more sophisticated than they used to be and may not cause complete numbness in the legs and feet.

When an epidural is given

Theoretically, you could have an epidural at any point during labour, even in the second stage when you are pushing your baby out, although a spinal injection (see p 172) would probably be offered in that situation. Most women tend to have an epidural when their cervix is about 5–6 cm dilated and their contractions are getting very strong. If you are as much as 8–9 cm dilated, your midwife may tell you that it's too late to have an epidural and advise you to manage without because your baby should be born soon.

The advantages

You might decide you want an epidural for the following reasons:

- More than 90 per cent of women who have an epidural get complete pain relief.
- You don't become drowsy with an epidural so your mind remains totally clear.
- It can help to control high blood pressure.
- Not having to deal with the pain may make you feel more in control and restore your confidence.

The disadvantages

You might decide against having an epidural for the following reasons:

- It will mean your labour is less active because your mobility is affected.
- You need to have a drip in your arm. This is because an epidural can cause a drop in blood pressure, affecting oxygen flow to your baby. With the drip the volume of blood can be boosted to bring your blood pressure back to normal.
- An epidural means you can't tell when you need to empty your bladder, so a catheter is used.
- You may have to be told when to push if the epidural hasn't worn off. Your midwife and doctor manage your labour for you.
- Epidurals can increase the length of labour.
- There's a greater chance of needing to have an assisted delivery (see pp 190–1).
- If the epidural needle goes beyond the epidural space, there will be a leakage of cerebro-spinal fluid after the tube is taken out. Even a very small leak will give you a terrible headache.
- Some women have problems passing urine after having an epidural.
- Not every hospital in England and Wales offers a 24-hour epidural service.
- Not available for a home birth.

HAVING THE INJECTION *You will be asked to sit on the edge of the bed and lean forward slightly, or you may be asked to lie on your side. Concentrate on your breathing. Breathe in deeply through your nose and slowly out through your mouth. Try to keep very still while the anaesthetist is setting up the epidural.*

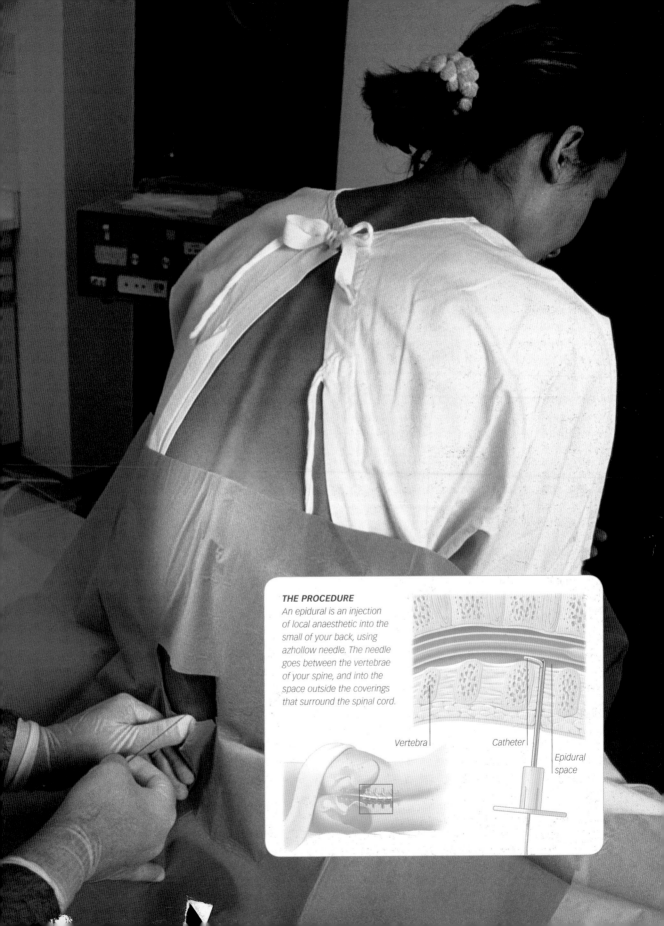

THE PROCEDURE

An epidural is an injection of local anaesthetic into the small of your back, using azhollow needle. The needle goes between the vertebrae of your spine, and into the space outside the coverings that surround the spinal cord.

Vertebra

Catheter

Epidural space

How will the position of my baby affect the labour and birth?

The way your baby is lying in your uterus can affect the progress and length of your labour. Ideally he will be head down and facing your spine. In any other position, medical intervention may be needed to deliver him safely.

What position would my baby ideally be in for the birth?

The best position is for your baby to be head down, with the back of his head slightly towards the front of your tummy. This is known as the anterior position. Labour is nearly always shorter and easier when your baby is in this position because he fits snugly into the curve of your pelvis and it's easy for him to move down during labour. When he gets to the bottom of your pelvis, he turns his head so that the widest part of his head is in the widest part of your pelvis. The back of his head can then slip underneath your pubic bone and, as he is born, his face sweeps across the perineum, which is the tissue between the back of the vagina and anus.

What is a posterior position?

This is when the baby is positioned with the back of his head towards the mother's spine. The close proximity between the baby's bony skull and the spine can be very uncomfortable, and the best position to labour in is on all fours. In this position, your baby drops away from your spine, helping relieve the backache. Your waters are more likely to break at the beginning of labour when your baby is in the posterior position. When your baby gets to the bottom of your pelvis, he'll need to turn 180 degrees to get into the best position for birth. This can take a while, or he may not turn at all. In this case, he will be born with his face looking up. Forceps or ventouse (see pp 190–1) may be needed.

Why are some babies posterior?

Lifestyle is thought to be a big factor. When you are sitting in your car, or in a chair watching TV or working at a computer for many hours, your pelvis is tipped backwards. This is always true if you are in a position where your knees are raised above the level of your pelvis. When your pelvis is tipped backwards, the heaviest part of your baby, which

ASK THE EXPERT
DR MAGGIE BLOTT
CONSULTANT OBSTETRICIAN

What is the most usual position for twins and does this affect the type of delivery?

In most single pregnancies, the baby is head-down, but twins can be positioned in many combinations, such as one head-down and one breech (see right) or both breech. One of the most common reasons for a Caesarean for twins is the babies' position. When the first baby is head-down, for example, doctors will usually do a vaginal delivery and also try to deliver the second baby vaginally, even if he is breech. Some doctors try to avoid a Caesarean by doing a series of manoeuvres to try to turn your baby (see right). Many doctors, aware of the evidence that breech babies sometimes do less well delivered vaginally, will recommend a Caesarean if the first baby is breech.

is the back of his head and his spine, will also tend to swing round to the back. So he ends up in a posterior position, lying against your spine. If your lifestyle involves a lot of upright activity, your baby is far more likely to go down into your pelvis in an anterior position because your pelvis is always tipped forwards. There are ways to encourage your baby into the anterior position (see p 155).

What is a breech position?

This means that your baby is in a bottom-down position. If this is your first baby, he will probably move and settle into a head-down position in your pelvis around the eighth month of pregnancy. When labour begins, about 96 per cent of babies are lying head down, but a few (about three per cent) will settle into a breech position.

What if my baby is still breech near to the due date?

According to the latest guidelines from the Royal College of Obstetricians and Gynaecologists, your doctor or midwife should offer you the chance to have your baby turned manually into a head down position. This process is called external cephalic version (ECV). If performed after 38 weeks, it's successful in about two thirds of cases. Sometimes, however, the baby refuses to budge.

If my baby stays in a breech position, does it mean I will have to have a Caesarean section?

Research suggests that breech babies do better if they are delivered by Caesarean. However, some very senior midwives and doctors have challenged this research. They feel that a normal birth is just as safe, provided that the midwife or doctor has the special skills needed to help a woman give birth to a breech baby. Sadly many doctors and midwives no longer have these skills.

If you want a vaginal birth, your doctor may be more likely to be supportive if you've given birth vaginally before and you don't have a history of giving birth to big babies. Before making a final decision, you and your doctor should evaluate your situation and discuss the possible risks and benefits together.

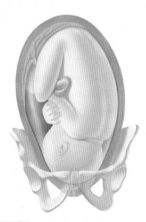

ANTERIOR
In this position the baby is head down with his back facing the mother's abdomen. This is the best position for an easy passage through the birth canal.

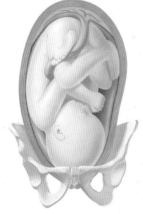

POSTERIOR
Here the baby is head down but his back is facing the mother's spine. This can cause back pain and a prolonged labour that may have to be assisted.

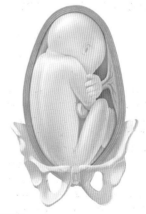

BREECH
When the baby doesn't turn head down, it is said to be breech. In a natural birth, the feet or buttocks would be delivered first, which requires a skilled midwife or doctor.

What happens in the first stage of labour?

The first stage of labour results in the neck of the uterus – the cervix – dilating to a full 10 cm and consists of early, active and transitional phases. You will spend the early stages of your labour at home. On arriving at hospital, the midwife will check how dilated you are and then keep a close eye on how your labour is progressing.

How will I know when I'm in labour?

You will feel your uterus starting to contract regularly. The contractions in the early phase help to soften the cervix, and this phase may last many hours. Some women may not even be aware of this early phase and are several centimetres dilated before they realize they're in labour. You are in active labour when your cervix has dilated, or opened, to 3–4 cm. Your contractions will be getting stronger, more frequent and longer in duration. Eventually they may come as frequently as every 3–4 minutes and last 60–90 seconds.

What should I do in the early stages?

You'll probably be able to potter around the house, go for a walk, watch television, take a warm bath or have a nap. Relax as much as you can. If you find the contractions are hard work, try using massage and relaxation techniques and experiment with positions that you find comfortable. If you want to use a TENS machine (see p 170), put it on during this early phase as it seems to work best when it is used from the very beginning of labour.

Try to work with your body. What is it telling you to do? Would you be more comfortable in a different position? Do you need a drink or some food to give you more energy? Would it help to go to the toilet? Do you need more information from your midwife to reassure you? Consider taking a warm shower or bath – warm water can really help ease the pain of labour. Or you may choose to use a birth pool (see p 170–1). Take care not to get over-tired before your labour is properly underway. If your contractions start at night, try to stay in bed and relax for as long as possible.

What, if anything, should I eat while I'm in labour?

It's nearly always best to be guided by what you feel like eating. However, it is worth remembering that meats and other high-fat foods can be heavy on the digestive system. Carbohydrates, such as bread, potatoes and rice, are especially good for labour because they guarantee a long, slow release of energy to help you through contractions. Sugary foods are easy to eat, and they do give you an energy boost, but the energy quickly dissipates and leaves you feeling quite low. Eat only as much as is comfortable; it's not a good idea to overload your stomach. Eating a snack every hour while

QUICK TIP

If your labour is slow, try a change of scenery; a short walk down the hospital corridor may help. Ask your midwife or partner to give you a massage to help you relax. Some women find that a good cry releases the emotional tension and helps them to 'let go'.

you're in early labour, before you go to the hospital or call the midwife, will store up plenty of energy for the work ahead. Once you're in strong labour, you will probably find that you don't want to eat much. Labour is thirsty work, and delivery rooms are usually very hot, so make sure you bring plenty of water to drink. Your birth companion might also want to take food and drink to the hospital as he or she is likely to be there for many hours.

What is transition and will the contractions change during this stage of labour?

Transition, or the transitional phase, is the last part of the first stage of labour, when the cervix dilates from 8 to 10 cm. During this phase of labour, contractions may last as long as 1–1½ minutes and occur every 2–3 minutes. They will feel stronger and more painful than the earlier ones. Hang on to the thought that you are nearly there and will soon meet your baby. Make the most of the time in between contractions to rest and relax. Keep your breathing as rhythmical as possible (breathe in through your nose and blow out through a soft mouth), and if you want to shout, groan and make a lot of noise, go for it!

> **JUST THE FACTS**
> THE BEST POSITIONS FOR LABOUR
>
> *You won't know which position will be the best for you until you're actually in labour. Listen to your body and choose a position that best helps you to cope with the contractions. You could:*
>
> - *Lean on a work surface or against the back of a chair.*
> - *Put your arms round your partner's neck or waist and lean on him.*
> - *Lean on the bed in the delivery room (with the height adjusted for your comfort) or against a window-sill.*
> - *Kneel on a large cushion or pillow on the floor and lean forwards onto the seat of a chair.*
> - *Sit astride a chair, resting on a pillow placed across the top.*
> - *Sit on the toilet, leaning forwards, or sit astride, leaning on the cistern.*
> - *Get on all fours.*
> - *Kneel on one leg with the other bent. Rock your hips backwards and forwards or in a circle to help your baby through your pelvis and to help you stay relaxed.*

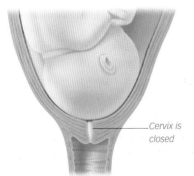

Cervix is closed

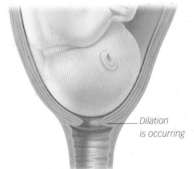

Dilation is occurring

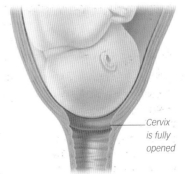

Cervix is fully opened

LATENT
The cervix is closed but begins to thin and soften – known as effacement. Once this has happened, your contractions will cause the cervix to dilate.

ACTIVE
The active stage starts when the cervix has dilated by at least 3–4 cm. The contractions will begin to be more intense and last for longer.

TRANSITION
This is the end of the third stage when the cervix dilates from 8 to 10 cm. Once it is fully dilated, you can begin to push your baby out.

What happens once I'm in hospital?

If you're having your baby in hospital the midwife will carry out some basic checks when you arrive. As well as monitoring your baby's heartbeat to ensure she isn't distressed, she will record the rate of your contractions. Ideally you will progress at a steady rate but if you don't, a method of speeding up labour may be offered.

What checks are carried out when I arrive at hospital?

If you are having your baby in hospital, many delivery suites have a special room for mothers who have just arrived. Here the midwife (whom you may or may not have met already) will ask you to tell her what has happened so far: for example, whether your waters have broken. She'll also need to see your maternity notes.

Your blood pressure, temperature, pulse and urine will be checked and the midwife will feel your tummy to find out which way round your baby is. She will ask your permission to do a vaginal examination to find out how many centimetres your cervix has dilated. The midwife records everything on a chart, called a partogram, so that if she goes off duty the next midwife will be able to see at a glance how your labour is progressing.

How will my baby be monitored?

Your baby's heartbeat may be monitored with a Sonicaid or ear trumpet, but sometimes electronic fetal monitoring is used. This procedure uses two electronic sensors that monitor your baby's heartbeat and your rate of contractions. By studying the relationship between the two, your midwife gets an idea of how your baby is coping with labour. It is only usually necessary if a pregnancy is high risk but you can ask to be monitored in this way if it makes you feel more secure.

The sensors are held in place with elastic belts. These can feel quite tight on your tummy so ask to have them loosened if you're very uncomfortable. Each sensor is attached to a wire, which in turn is attached to a machine. Sometimes, a small clip is placed on your baby's head and this, rather than the abdominal sensor, monitors her heartbeat.

If your baby's heartbeat is being monitored with a Sonicaid or an ear trumpet, your midwife just needs to be able to get at the right part of your abdomen, which she can easily do whatever your position. If you have to be monitored using electronic sensors, ask if you can sit in a chair. This is much more comfortable than lying on a bed for hours and allows you to be more active.

ASK THE EXPERT
CHRISSIE HAMMONDS
MIDWIFE SONOGRAPHER

How will my baby be monitored if I'm in a birth pool during labour?

If you're in a bath or birth pool, your baby's heartbeat can be monitored using a special waterproof Sonicaid called an Aqua-aid. All you have to do is lift your tummy to the surface of the water when the midwife wants to check the heartbeat. If she thinks your baby is having problems, she'll ask you to get out of the pool to be monitored using the electronic sensors for a short while. If everything is progressing well, you'll then be able to get back into the pool.

How long will labour last?

Mothers generally time labour from when they feel the first contraction, or their waters break. However, midwives and doctors calculate the length of labour from when the cervix is 3–4 cm dilated. This is considered to be the start of the 'active phase' of labour (see p 178). By this point, you might have been having quite painful tightening for some hours and feel as though you have been in labour for quite a long time already. Once your cervix is 3 cm dilated, you can expect it to be about 8–14 hours until your baby is born. Women who have given birth before often have shorter labours than women giving birth for the first time, but individual cases do vary. It's not necessarily better for either you or your baby if labour is quick. In fact, very fast labours can be physically and emotionally draining.

Why might labour be slow?

For all sorts of reasons. Some labours are slow because the mother is very tense. Labour might also be slow because of the baby's position, because the contractions are not very strong, or because the mother's pelvis is not quite the right shape or size for the baby's head to easily fit into. During labour the baby's head is gradually moulded by the contractions as they push the baby further down into the pelvis, and it's better for the baby if this happens slowly. It usually takes much longer for the cervix to open up the first five centimetres than the second five. This is because, as the contractions get stronger, they open up the cervix more quickly.

Can labour be speeded up?

Labour is occasionally so slow that there's a real risk of the mother and baby becoming exhausted. Augmentation – the speeding up of labour – may be recommended if the contractions are becoming

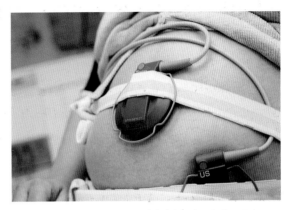

ELECTRONIC MONITORING *Your baby's heartbeat and your contractions may be recorded using electronic fetal monitoring. This can be more restricting because you're hooked up to a machine, but you can ask to be seated rather than lie on a bed.*

weaker and further apart, and there is little or no progress in the rate at which your cervix is dilating. If the doctor or midwife breaks your waters, this may be enough to get labour going again, or you may have a drip put into a vein in your arm to stimulate contractions (see p 189). Your baby's heartbeat will need to be continuously monitored to make sure she is not getting stressed with the increase in the strength and frequency of contractions. The drip will also contain sugars and salts, which will give you more energy.

JUST THE FACTS
NATURAL WAYS TO SPEED UP LABOUR

Contractions may open up the cervix more quickly and therefore lead to a shorter labour if you:

- *Are upright and regularly change your position.*
- *Eat and drink as and when you need to in order to maintain energy levels.*
- *Go to the toilet regularly – a full bladder can slow your labour down and a walk to the toilet can speed it up.*
- *Relax – try inhaling a drop of lavender oil on a handkerchief or listen to some soothing music.*

What happens in the second stage of labour?

Once your cervix has dilated to 10 cm, the work and excitement of the second stage of labour begin. This is when your baby is pushed down the birth canal into the world. It can feel like very hard work, but as you begin to feel your baby emerge you'll know that the end is in sight.

How will I know when I'm in the second stage of labour?

There's often a lull at the end of the first stage when the contractions stop and you and your baby can rest for a while. When the contractions start again, you'll feel the pressure of your baby's head between your legs. With each contraction and every push, your baby will move down your pelvis a little, but at the end of the contraction, he'll slip back up again! Don't despair. As long as the baby keeps on moving down a little each time, you're doing fine. When your baby's head is far down in your pelvis and stretching the opening of the vagina, you may feel a hot, stinging sensation and your midwife will tell you that your baby's head has 'crowned'.

As your baby's head begins to emerge, she may ask you to stop pushing and tell you to gently pant. This helps make sure that your baby is born gently and slowly, and should reduce the risk of you tearing. If you have had a baby before, the second stage may only take 5–10 minutes. If this is your first baby, it may take an hour or more.

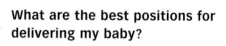

ASK THE EXPERT
CHRISSIE HAMMONDS
MIDWIFE SONOGRAPHER

What is an episiotomy and why might it be necessary to have one?

An episiotomy is a surgical cut in the perineum, the muscular area between the vagina and the back passage. A local anaesthetic to numb the perineum is given beforehand. Your midwife might suggest one if your baby is becoming distressed and needs to be born quickly, or if she thinks that you may tear badly unless the opening of the vagina is enlarged. Some health professionals believe that an episiotomy heals better than a tear, although research doesn't back this up. Spontaneous tears are less painful or at least no more painful in the days after the birth than episiotomies. Research suggests that episiotomies may actually result in more pain, incontinence and poor healing, with few benefits. If your doctor or midwife suggests an episiotomy, do make sure that they explain fully why it is necessary.

What are the best positions for delivering my baby?

Your baby will find it easier to be born if you are in an upright position because you will be able to bear down more efficiently. The combination of the muscular action of the uterus, your pushing efforts and gravity is a powerful one. If the midwife prefers you to give birth on the bed, kneel on the mattress and lean against a large pile of pillows placed at the top end. Or put your arms round your partner's neck as he stands at the bedside. If your midwife is happy for you to give birth on the floor, try kneeling. When the time comes for your baby's head to be born, all fours is an excellent position. Because gravity is not so effective in this position, your baby's head is able to emerge very gently from the vagina, reducing your risk of tearing. The squatting position has also been shown to increase the outlet

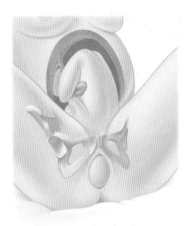

BABY'S HEAD CROWNS
To begin with your baby's head will be visible but will keep slipping back inside the vagina. Once it remains visible, you will be told your baby's head has 'crowned'.

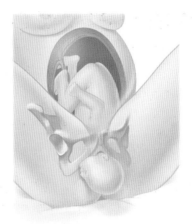

HEAD EMERGES
Your baby's head will emerge and the midwife will check that the umbilical cord isn't wrapped around his neck. You may be asked to pant to prevent tearing.

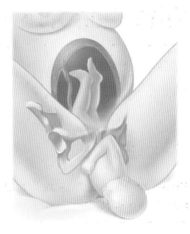

BABY IS BORN
Although your baby emerges face down, his head will turn to one side. With a couple more contractions his shoulders and his body will slide out.

through the pelvis compared to lying on your back, so it is a good one to try if you have been pushing for a while without much progress.

How do I manage to push and breathe at the same time during the second stage?

Take a deep breath when you feel your contraction starting, and then breathe or blow out slowly as you bear down. This will prevent you from damaging your throat, ensure that you maintain a healthy breathing pattern and result in effective pushing. If you have had an epidural, and can't feel where you are meant to be pushing, take a deep breath when your midwife tells you there is a contraction beginning, and as you blow out, let your mind travel down your body to between your legs, and push.

Sometimes women are advised to hold their breath and push for as long as possible. This is not a good idea. You will deprive yourself and your baby of oxygen, and you'll quickly exhaust yourself. You should push as many times per contraction as feels right – this is usually about four or five pushes for every contraction.

Why are women sometimes advised not to push?

It can be difficult not to push when nature is telling you to, but if the neck of the womb doesn't open up evenly, leaving a 'lip' of cervix round your baby's head, you may be advised not to. Try positioning yourself with your face on the floor and your bottom in the air and panting through your contractions. This can tip the baby off the cervix and should reduce your desire to push. If you've had an epidural, your midwife will tell you when to push. She may wait until she can see your baby's head.

IF YOU DO NOTHING ELSE...

- *Remember childbirth is natural – try to relax and listen to your body.*
- *Talk to your midwife throughout and ask her to explain what is happening.*
- *Keep in mind the end result – your beautiful newborn baby.*

What happens in the third stage of labour?

In the third stage of labour, the placenta is delivered along with the membranes that surrounded your baby. This can occur naturally or, alternatively, can be helped along with an injection of a synthetic hormone. This helps to stimulate contractions and speed up the rate at which the placenta separates from the wall of the uterus.

What happens after your baby is born?

Contractions will resume for a few minutes, but won't be as intense. These cause the placenta to peel away and drop into the bottom of your uterus. The placenta, with the membranes of the empty bag of waters attached, will pass down and out of your vagina. Your midwife will carefully examine the placenta and membranes to make sure nothing has been left behind. She will feel your tummy to check that your uterus is contracting to stop the bleeding from the place where the placenta was attached. You may hardly be aware of the third stage, as your focus has probably shifted to your baby.

How quickly is the placenta delivered?

Delivering the placenta usually takes from 5–15 minutes, but it can take up to an hour. It depends on whether you have a managed or natural third stage (see right). Most women are surprised at how much easier it is to deliver the placenta than to push the baby out. You may like to have a look at it.

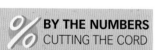

BY THE NUMBERS
CUTTING THE CORD

Dads, did you cut your baby's umbilical cord?

56% *Yes.*
44% *No.*

Source: Based on a BabyCentre.co.uk poll of 3,372 dads.

What is a natural third stage?

A physiological or natural third stage means that you wait for the placenta to be delivered naturally. This may take up to an hour to happen, though skin-to-skin contact and breastfeeding your baby will help the uterus to start contracting. You need to actively help the delivery of the placenta by pushing with contractions, perhaps in the squatting position. Cord clamping can be left until after the cord has stopped pulsating, so that your baby gets more oxygenated blood from the placenta. There is usually more blood loss with a physiological third stage, so it is not advisable if you have had any complications of the pregnancy such as anaemia, heavy bleeding or high blood pressure, a twin pregnancy, an induced or very long labour, or an assisted delivery.

What is a managed third stage?

A managed third stage means you have an injection in your thigh just as your baby is being born which causes the uterus to contract strongly to deliver the placenta quickly. You do not have to push or do anything as the midwife will wait until your uterus is contracted, and then pull gently on the cord to deliver the placenta. The cord will be clamped soon after the baby is born. The advantage of this method is that it is over quickly and there is little blood loss. The disadvantage is that the drugs used may make

THE FIRST FEED *If you're going to breastfeed, offer the breast as soon as possible – your midwife will help you. This can help to speed up natural delivery of the placenta. Don't worry if your baby doesn't seem very interested. Even if she's only touching and nuzzling you, it can help to stimulate contractions and establish feeding patterns.*

you feel sick or faint, or give you a headache. There is also a small chance that the placenta may get trapped inside the uterus if the cervix closes before it is delivered.

What happens next?

The midwife will examine your perineum (the area of skin between your vagina and back passage) and vagina to see if you need any stitches. This is always necessary after an episiotomy (see p 182) or deep tear. If you had an epidural, this can be topped up so you don't feel any discomfort. If you haven't had an epidural, you'll be given an injection of local anaesthetic. Tell the midwife if it is sore while she is putting in the stitches and she can give you more anaesthetic. Small tears and grazes are usually left to heal on their own. Lastly the midwife will help you to wash and freshen up.

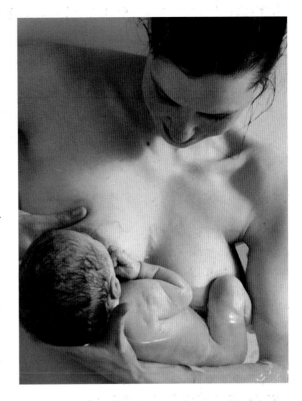

How am I likely to feel in the first hour of the birth?

You may feel shaky due to adrenaline and the adjustments that your body immediately starts to make. It's also common to feel very hungry. Some women are on a high, and can't wait to crack open the champagne and tell the world about their new arrival. However, others find it hard to pay attention to the baby if they have had a long labour, or if they've had pethidine (see p 172). There's nothing wrong with their maternal instincts; they're simply exhausted. If this happens to you, give yourself time. You'll feel much better and more interested in your baby when you've had some rest.

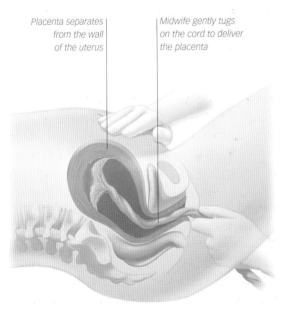

Placenta separates from the wall of the uterus

Midwife gently tugs on the cord to deliver the placenta

DELIVERY OF THE PLACENTA *The umbilical cord will lengthen, indicating that the placenta has separated from the uterus. The midwife will gently tug on it to deliver the placenta; it usually comes away quickly and easily.*

What checks will be carried out on my newborn baby?

Whether your baby is born in hospital or at home, he will be assessed using a method known as the Apgar scale. This quick check, which is carried out by your midwife straight after the birth, is a reliable indicator of any health problems.

What will my newborn look like?

Few newborns are beauty contest contenders, which isn't surprising considering what they've just been through. They have big heads, no necks, short legs and big, distended torsos. Because newborns have spent an average of 12 hours squeezing through the birth canal, their head can often be misshapen, with a pointy appearance. Babies born by Caesarean actually have an edge beauty-wise, because their heads don't have to squeeze through the birth canal. But as funny-looking as your newborn may seem, you'll soon be convinced that your child is the most beautiful baby ever born.

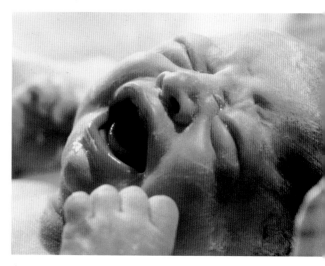

I'VE ARRIVED! Your baby may be born covered in vernix and blood and is likely to have a red and wrinkled face. All this is perfectly normal, though, given what he's been through. He'll soon let you know from his first cry that everything is in good working order.

BabyCentre Buzz

"I'm 38 weeks pregnant and know that I'm expecting a boy. I just cannot stop thinking about what he will look like. I just wish I knew!" Carol

"My third baby was a peculiar sight when he was born. His hands and feet were a ghostly white, while his face and the rest of his body went through every colour of the rainbow. Still, within five minutes he looked just as precious and handsome as his brothers." Ali

"My baby came out well-cooked...he was beautiful and wrinkle-free. He had a cone-shaped head, but that quickly went away." Vicki

I've been told my baby will be assessed using the Apgar scale. What is it?

This is a simple and effective method used to measure your newborn's health and to determine if he needs any quick treatment. It is quick, painless, and very reassuring. At one minute and again at five minutes after birth, your baby is evaluated for heart rate, respiration, muscle tone, reflex response and skin colour.

Each factor is given a score between zero and two (see right) then the scores are added up. Most newborns score between 7 and 10 and don't need immediate treatment. If your newborn does require medical help, it is much better to be aware of this straightaway.

What do the Apgar scores mean?

A 'perfect 10' is music to proud parents' ears, but an eight or a nine is still good news. A difficult delivery, premature birth or pain medication can artificially suppress the score so that the Apgar doesn't depict your baby's true condition, but generally babies who score between 8 and 10 are in good to excellent condition and usually need only routine care. Those who score between 5 and 7 are in fair condition and may require some help breathing. Your midwife may vigorously rub the baby's skin or give him a whiff of oxygen. Babies who score under five may be in poor condition and require some help. Your baby would be placed on a trolley in the delivery room. This has heat, light and oxygen to warm him up and help him to breathe. A paediatrician will be called to check him over.

What other checks are needed?

The midwife will examine your baby to make sure everything looks normal – she will feel the roof of his mouth to make sure there is no cleft, and count his fingers and toes. Your baby will be weighed and measured. If you are in hospital, an identification band will be put on your baby's wrist and ankle. Your baby may also, with your permission, be given vitamin K to protect against bleeding.

What are fontanelles?

These are the two soft spots on your baby's skull, which during labour allow the head to compress enough to fit through the birth canal. The rear fontanelle takes about four months to close, while the front one takes between 9 and 18 months.

JUST THE FACTS
APGAR SCORE

An Apgar score of between 0 and 2 is assigned for each check, with 10 being the highest possible total score (see left).

Heart rate
0: No heart rate.
1: Fewer than 100 beats a minute.
2: More than 100 beats a minute.

Respiration
0: Not breathing.
1: Weak cry or slow, irregular breathing.
2: Good, strong cry.

Muscle tone
0: Limp.
1: Some bending of arms and legs.
2: Active motion.

Reflex response
0: No response to airways being suctioned.
1: Grimace during suctioning.
2: Grimace and cough or sneeze during suctioning.

Colour
0: The baby's whole body is completely blue or pale.
1: Good colour in body but blue hands or feet.
2: Completely pink (for dark-skinned babies, pink on palms, soles, lips and mouth).

When will I be able to hold and feed my newborn baby?

You may choose to have your newborn delivered straight on to your bare tummy. Called 'skin to skin' this is a lovely way for you and your baby to start the bonding process. If you like, you can let him breastfeed straight away, or you may want him wrapped in a towel before you feed him for the first time. If you are bottlefeeding, you can feed him as soon as you are both ready.

If you've had a Caesarean delivery (see pp 192–3), your newborn baby will usually be given to your partner to hold .

Why and how is labour induced?

Most labours begin naturally at some time between 39 and 41 weeks of pregnancy. If this doesn't happen, you may be 'induced', which means your labour is started by artificial means. Labour can also be speeded up if it started spontaneously, but the cervix is not dilating because of weak contractions.

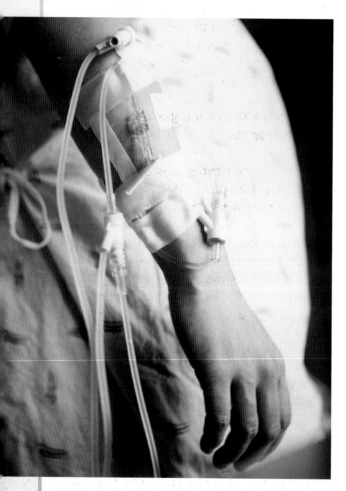

ARTIFICIAL HORMONES *If other methods of induction are ineffective, Syntocinon, an artificial hormone, may be given through an intravenous drip – it goes into your bloodstream through a tiny tube into a vein in your arm. Once contractions have begun, the rate of the drip can be adjusted so that contractions occur often enough to make your cervix dilate, without becoming too powerful.*

What happens if I'm overdue?

If you are overdue you will go for an antenatal appointment at 41 weeks. The midwife will check that your due date is correct, by confirming when you had your last period, whether your cycle normally lasts 28 days and referring to your early ultrasound scan if you had one. She will examine your tummy to check the position and size of your baby and, with your permission, she may carry out an internal examination to see whether your cervix feels ready for labour (that is, soft and stretchy). She may offer to sweep your membranes (see right) to trigger labour. Finally, she will discuss inducing your baby. If you decide upon induction, you will be given a date to come into hospital when you are 42 weeks pregnant.

In what circumstances is labour induced?

Although it's usually best to let nature take its course, sometimes the birth process may need a little help. Labour is induced when the risks of prolonging your pregnancy are more serious than the risks of delivering your baby right away. If you are more than two weeks overdue there is a slightly increased risk of late stillbirth and induction is offered to reduce this risk. If you have a medical condition such as diabetes or pre-eclampsia (see p 135) or you have previously had a stillborn baby you may need to be induced earlier than 42 weeks.

BabyCentre Buzz

"I maintained that if I set my sights on my baby being born two weeks late, I wouldn't become so despondent." Penny

"Every twinge and movement you think 'this is it' but alas no..." Mandana

"If there is some medical reason for having an induction then take that advice, but don't feel pushed into it. Make an informed decision." Sara

Do I have to be induced if my waters have broken?

Not necessarily, but the risk of infection grows the longer the waters have been broken. Research shows that 70 per cent of mothers give birth within 24 hours, and almost 90 per cent within 72 hours, of their waters breaking. So you could opt to wait for labour to begin, or you could choose to be induced. In either case, your midwife and doctor will observe you closely for any signs of infection.

How is labour induced?

You may be given a membrane sweep in which the membranes that surround your baby are separated from your cervix. This is carried out during an internal examination. It's been shown to be effective in stimulating labour and is now offered routinely to women who are overdue before any other methods of induction. It can be uncomfortable if the cervix is difficult to reach and can occasionally cause a bit of bleeding.

Another method is to insert a pessary or gel containing prostaglandin into the vagina. Prostaglandin is a hormone-like substance, which helps stimulate contractions.

Sometimes the waters will be artificially broken, known as artificially rupturing the membranes (ARM). A long thin probe, which looks a little like a fine crochet hook, is passed through your cervix and makes a small break in the membranes around your baby. This procedure is often effective when the cervix feels soft and ready for labour to start. If labour doesn't start following these techniques, or if your contractions are not very effective, Syntocinon – a synthetic form of the hormone oxytocin – may be given through a drip. You may be offered an epidural (see pp 174–5) for pain relief because with Syntocinon the contractions can be intense from the outset.

What are the disadvantages of being given Syntocinon?

Syntocinon can cause strong contractions and put your baby under stress, so you'll need continuous electronic monitoring (see pp 180-1). The contractions brought on by Syntocinon are often more painful than natural ones, so you're also more likely to want medical pain relief. You're more likely to need an assisted delivery (see pp 190–1) following an induction, or a Caesarean. This may be due to complications in the pregnancy that led to the induction or it may be due to problems caused by the induction itself.

IF YOU DO NOTHING ELSE...

- *Remember that you have a choice about whether or not to have your baby induced.*
- *Talk to your midwife and doctors about the methods they're proposing to use.*
- *Think about what pain relief you might use because the contractions following an induction using Syntocinon can be difficult to cope with.*

What is an assisted delivery?

An assisted delivery is when either forceps or ventouse are used to help your baby be born. Both are instruments that are attached to the baby's head so that he can be pulled out. Your baby may need assistance for various reasons, including if he becomes distressed or if you are no longer able to push.

What happens in a forceps delivery?

Forceps are sometimes described as 'stainless steel salad servers' or 'large sugar-tongs'. They come in two intersecting parts, and have curved ends to cradle the baby's head. You'll be asked to put your legs in stirrups or supports at the side of the bed and the end of the bed will be removed. A thin tube called a catheter, attached to a bag, will be put into your bladder to empty it and your legs will be draped in sheets. Your doctor will need to make a cut known as an episiotomy (see p 182) through the back of your vagina to enlarge the opening and prevent excessive tearing.

> **JUST THE FACTS**
> REASONS FOR ASSISTED DELIVERY
>
> *Your midwife and doctor might discuss a forceps or ventouse delivery with you if:*
>
> - *Your baby has become distressed during the second (pushing) stage of labour.*
> - *You are very tired and can no longer push.*
> - *Your baby isn't making any progress through your pelvis.*
> - *There's a medical reason why you shouldn't push for too long (for example, you suffer from heart disease).*
> - *You are having twins and need help delivering your second baby.*

What happens in a ventouse delivery?

The ventouse has a cup attached to a small vacuum pump. The cup, which fits on top and slightly towards the back of your baby's head, may be made of metal or silicone plastic. The soft cups are less likely to cause damage to your baby's head, but the metal cups are less likely to slip off.

You will be asked to put your legs in supports. The ventouse cup will be placed on the baby's head inside the vagina, and then the air is sucked out of the cup using a foot-controlled vacuum pump or a hand-held pump. This can be noisy, so be prepared. Once the cup is securely fixed, the doctor will ask you to push with your next contraction, and then he or she will pull on the cup to help your baby out. Occasionally, the cup comes off the baby's head, especially if the baby is large or in a position where the cup does not fix well, and has to be reapplied. If the baby is in a position that makes delivery more difficult, then a metal cup or semi-rigid plastic cup ventouse may be used because these are less likely to come off.

Is ventouse preferable to forceps?

Nowadays, many doctors prefer to use the ventouse for assisted deliveries. This is because the ventouse is less painful for the mother both during and after the birth. There's less risk of your bladder or bowel function being damaged than with forceps, and you

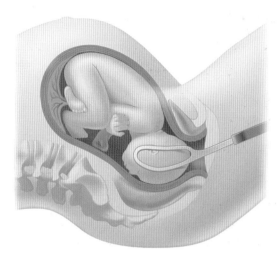

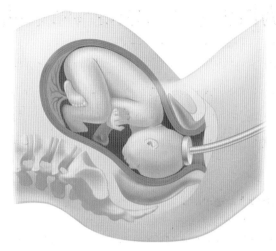

FORCEPS DELIVERY
The 'tongs' of the forceps are placed around the baby's head.
The doctor will then pull on the forceps while you push during
a contraction. Forceps are safe instruments but may cause
some temporary bruising on your baby's head.

VENTOUSE DELIVERY
This is a suction device that is attached to the baby's head.
The doctor will pull on the cup as you push during a contraction.
Ventouse is safe but it may cause your baby's head to be slightly
misshapen for a few days.

might not have to have an episiotomy (see p 182). It used to be said that a baby could be delivered faster using forceps than ventouse, but research shows that this isn't true.

Will an assisted delivery affect my baby?

With a forceps delivery, your baby may be slightly bruised, but this clears up in a few days. Very occasionally the facial nerve is temporarily damaged, causing the baby's mouth to droop at one corner. Babies sometimes have cone-shaped heads for a couple of days after a ventouse delivery. A blood blister may form on top of the baby's head, but this usually disappears in a week; your baby's head may also be slightly grazed. It's usual for a paediatrician to attend an assisted birth.

How will an assisted delivery affect me?

Most forceps births are straightforward, although you may experience some soreness and bruising afterwards. You may find it difficult to pass urine, or

may leak urine when you're not on the toilet, or you may develop constipation. Your midwife will be able to advise you on these problems. The risk of injury is greater with forceps than with ventouse delivery as are reports of severe pain in the perineum (the area between the vagina and anus).

Occasionally there may be a tear into the back passage, known as a third degree tear. These tears need to be repaired in the operating theatre. To allow the tear time to heal, it's important to avoid constipation so you'll be given a laxative for a few days. The majority of these tears heal well and there are no later problems, but in rare cases there is permanent damage to the back passage or bladder.

IF YOU DO NOTHING ELSE...

Make sure you understand the reasons why an assisted delivery was necessary, or you could find yourself worrying whether you'll need to have forceps or ventouse again when you come to give birth to your next baby.

What happens during a Caesarean?

A Caesarean is an operation in which your baby is lifted out of your abdomen rather than delivered naturally through your vagina. While it is a quick and effective procedure, it must be remembered that it is major surgery and does carry more risks than a natural birth. It will also mean a longer period of recovery for you.

How is the baby delivered?

The obstetrician will make an incision through your abdomen and uterus and remove your baby through it. A small horizontal incision (called a bikini cut) is made above the pubic bone, and then a second cut is made in the lower section of the uterus. The baby is then lifted out. The whole procedure only takes a few minutes. Your baby will be quickly checked over by a paediatrician and then shown to you. If

your baby is very small or unwell she may need to go straight to the Special Care Baby Unit. Otherwise your partner can hold her while the placenta is delivered and you are stitched up. This takes about 30 minutes. Each layer of muscle and skin needs to be closed using stitches.

Will I remain conscious during the birth?

Most Caesarean births are done with an epidural or spinal injection (see p 172) so you can be awake and see your baby immediately after the birth. As well as the epidural in your back, you will have a catheter inserted to drain your bladder, and a drip in your arm or hand to give extra fluids. You may also have a heart monitor on. A screen will be put up while the procedure is taking place. Your partner can stay with you during most of the preparation, and for the birth. Some partners like to peek over the screen but others prefer not to see what is happening. Only when your Caesarean is a true emergency, or if you need a general anaesthetic, will your partner be asked to leave.

How can I minimize my chances of having a Caesarean?

Many Caesareans save the life of the mother or baby, or both, so not all can be avoided. But there are some ways that you may be able to reduce your chances of having one, including staying healthy

ASK THE EXPERT
DR MAGGIE BLOTT
CONSULTANT OBSTETRICIAN

My first two babies were born by Caesarean. Is it safe to have another for my third child?

It used to be thought that if you had one Caesarean delivery you had to have the rest of your babies that way. However, this is no longer the case. Vaginal birth after a previous Caesarean – known as VBAC – is now common and safe. Current thinking also appears to be that a Caesarean should only be done for a good reason as, like any form of major surgery, it is never without risks. However, if another Caesarean is your only option for the delivery of your baby, your consultant will give you individual advice on the health of your uterus and the safety for you of another operation. There are many things that need to be considered, including your weight, age, medical history, fertility history and childbirth history, as well as personal choice. The reasons why you needed your previous Caesareans will also be considered.

so that you are in optimum condition for labour. Also find out what the Caesarean rates are locally. If you have a choice of hospitals, check the rates at each and compare them. Booking your care with a midwife can help since fewer women with midwifery-led care need a Caesarean. Studies show that the presence of a trained, supportive doula (see p 148) during delivery can also reduce the incidence of Caesareans. Your mobility during labour is also a factor: choosing an upright position can cut the length of labour.

How long should I wait after a Caesarean section before getting pregnant again?

The traditional advice used to be that women should have no more than three Caesareans and that they should wait a year after one before becoming pregnant again. Many obstetricians still

A FAMILY AFFAIR Your partner is usually allowed to stay in the delivery room throughout and can even watch the procedure if he wishes. Unless your baby needs special care, he will be allowed to hold her immediately after the birth and show her to you.

> **JUST THE FACTS**
> REASONS FOR AN EMERGENCY CAESAREAN
>
> *An emergency Caesarean might be necessary for the following reasons:*
> - *Your baby's heart rate becomes irregular.*
> - *The umbilical cord prolapses, or slips, through the cervix.*
> - *The placenta has abrupted (come adrift).*
> - *Your baby is not moving down the birth canal for any reason.*

stick to this advice, but some feel that, for many women, the advice is over-cautious. In the vast majority of Caesareans, the incision into the uterus is made horizontally into the lower segment of the uterus. These incisions usually heal well and are thought to be fully healed in three months. Nevertheless, many women underestimate the effect that a Caesarean will have on them. It is, after all, a surgical procedure.

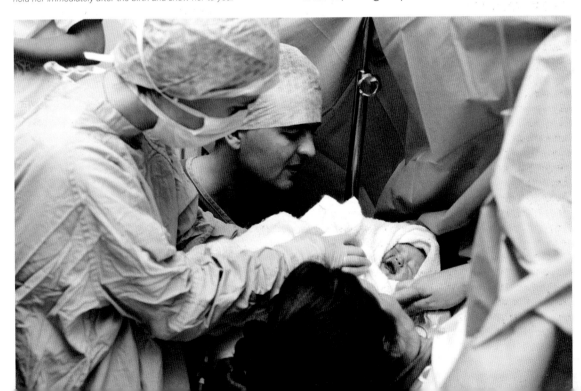

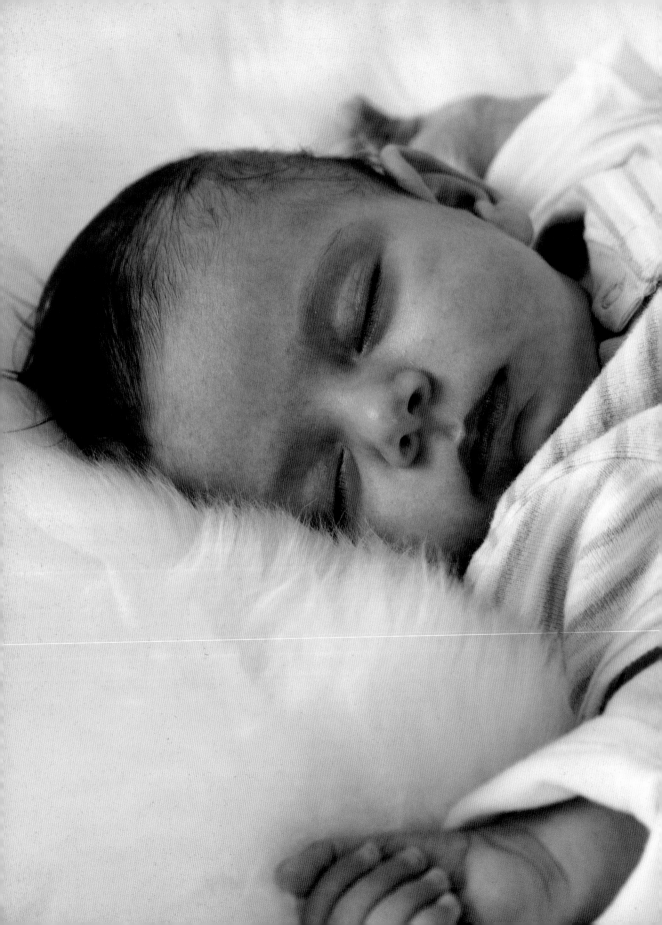

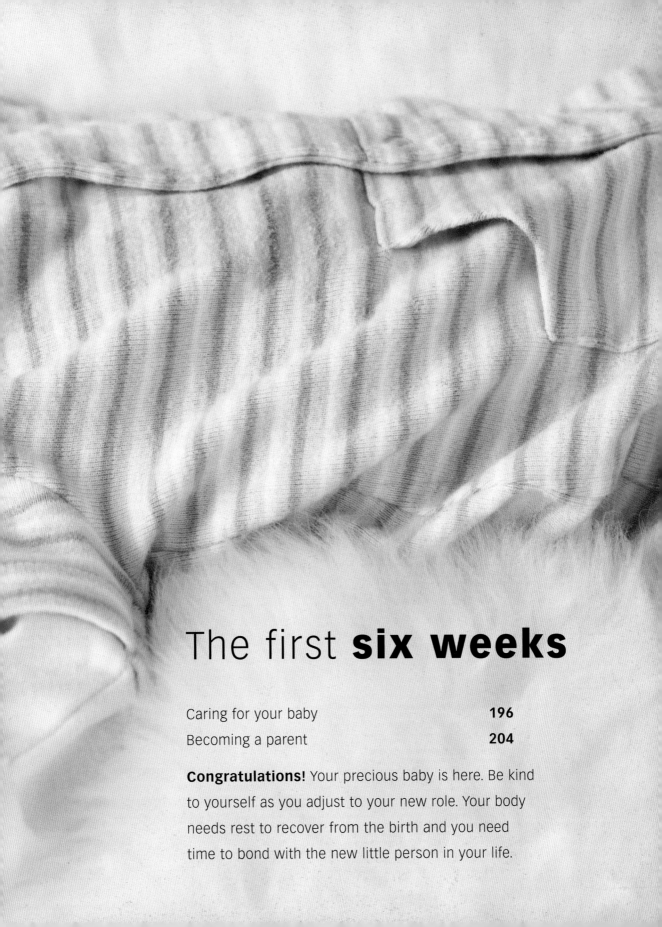

The first **six weeks**

Congratulations! Your precious baby is here. Be kind to yourself as you adjust to your new role. Your body needs rest to recover from the birth and you need time to bond with the new little person in your life.

How do I care for my newborn baby?

Looking after your newborn baby may be daunting, especially if you're a first-time parent. Remember that your midwife will continue to care for you and your baby for 10 days after the birth; you will then have access to a health visitor. Always seek advice if you are unsure about any aspect of your newborn's care.

When will my newborn baby's umbilical stump drop off?

The umbilical stump should dry up and drop off within 10–21 days, leaving a small wound that may take a few days to heal. The stump must be kept clean and dry, so when you're putting your baby's nappy on, fold it below the stump to expose it to the air and not to urine. Avoid bathing your baby until the area heals over completely, usually about 7–10 days after the birth. Sometimes, when the umbilical stump takes a long time to heal, bits of lumpy flesh – a type of connective tissue – appear in the wound. These are not a cause for concern and will soon disappear.

In the past, cord stumps have been cleaned with antiseptic tissues or an antiseptic powder, but recent studies have shown that leaving well alone helps the cord to heal. Consult your midwife if your baby develops a fever or appears unwell, if the navel and surrounding area become swollen or red, or if pus appears at the base of the stump.

ASK THE EXPERT
DAPHNE METLAND
BABYCENTRE EDITOR-IN-CHIEF

My newborn baby boy has jaundice. Is this common and how is it treated?

Yes, more than half of all healthy newborns develop a yellowish tinge to their skin. Jaundice develops in a healthy baby when the blood contains excess bilirubin – a chemical produced during the normal breakdown of old red blood cells. If your baby was born at term and is otherwise healthy, most doctors won't suggest treatment unless his bilirubin level is particularly high.

Jaundice is treated with phototherapy, where babies are exposed to fluorescent-type lights that break down excess bilirubin so it can be excreted through the baby's liver. The baby usually lies naked under the lights for a day or two, with his eyes covered by a mask. If your baby doesn't require phototherapy, you can help by giving him a little exposure to sunlight in the early morning or late afternoon. Frequent breastfeeds help as well.

How often do I need to change my newborn's nappy?

Change your newborn baby's nappies frequently; expect to do it before or after every feed (except at night, when nappy-changing may disrupt your baby's sleep) or when your baby has done a poo. Babies wee as often as every one to three hours and urine combined with bacteria in faeces can make a baby's skin sore and lead to nappy rash, so frequent changing is important.

Wetness doesn't bother most babies, so don't expect your baby to cry or show discomfort every time he needs changing. Disposables – especially the 'super-absorbent' ones – absorb moisture well, so you may not always be able to gauge the wetness until the nappy is oversaturated and more

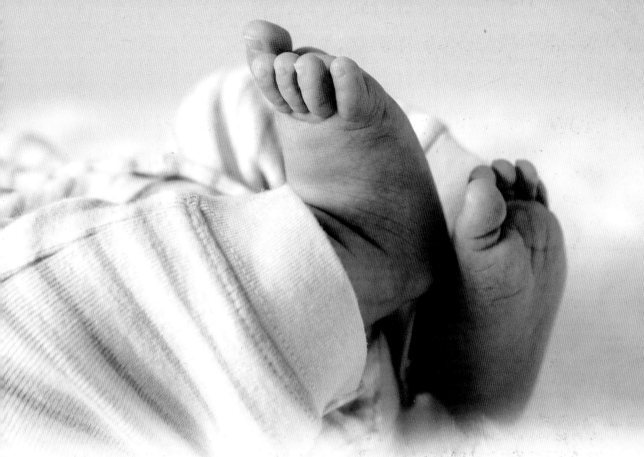

likely to cause real discomfort to your baby. To avoid the problem, check for wetness every couple of hours by rooting around a bit with a clean finger.

What causes nappy rash and what can I do to prevent it?

The main cause of nappy rash is wetness. Newborns wee often and have frequent, loose bowel movements. Even the most absorbent nappy leaves some moisture on a baby's delicate new skin. A baby left in a wet nappy for too long is more likely to develop nappy rash; however, it can still strike the bottoms of babies with particularly sensitive skin, even if their parents change the nappies frequently. Older babies who are sick and taking antibiotics may get diarrhoea, which can cause nappy rash.

The best remedy is to keep your baby clean and dry by changing his nappy frequently. If the weather is warm and he can play outside or in a room with an easy-clean floor, leave his nappy off for as long as possible to allow the air to speed up the healing process. You might also try switching disposable nappies and detergents to fragrance and additive-free brands: they'll probably clear up the problem if the nappy rash is allergy-based. Normal nappy rash should clear up after 3–4 days of at-home treatment. If it persists, try using an anti-yeast cream for a few days or seek the advice of your midwife or health visitor.

How often should I bath my baby?

You really only need to bath a newborn once or twice a week. Babies just don't get that dirty until they start crawling around. Use a gentle bath product suitable for babies or just plain water, and don't fill the baby bath too much. Some babies love their bath and enjoy the water, others scream throughout. Be guided by your baby. Instead of bathing your baby, you can 'top and tail' him. Use separate pieces of cotton wool dipped in warm water to clean his face and nappy area.

How can I make sure I get breastfeeding my baby off to a good start?

You can't prepare your nipples for the experience of breastfeeding, but you can prepare your mind. It helps to learn about breastfeeding before you start. Your partner should learn about it too, so that he can support and encourage you.

How should I position myself to breastfeed my baby?

Since feeds can take anything from 10–40 minutes, pick a comfortable place for breastfeeding. Have plenty of pillows and a drink and a snack to hand. You may want the telephone and the TV remote within reach as well. Make sure your feet are flat on the ground; if you are on tiptoes, your legs may tire. Remember to bring your baby up to your breast rather than lean over her, which may give you backache. Put a pillow or two under her to bring her up to the right height. Then turn her whole body so that she is facing you; it's almost impossible for

her to swallow if she has to turn her head to one side. Now position her so that her nose is just about facing your nipple. Touch her top lip lightly with your nipple then, as she opens her mouth wide, slip the nipple and a good mouthful of breast into her mouth. You do need to wait for her to open her mouth wide; if she only opens it a little, she will end up with your nipple clamped between her gums, which will make your nipples very sore (see left). If she's well latched on, your nipple will be right inside her mouth between her soft palate and her tongue. Once your baby latches on properly, she will be able to do the rest.

How often should I breastfeed?

Most newborns want to breastfeed 8–15 times a day in the first few days after the birth. Feed your baby as often as she needs it. Routines have no place in your day while you're getting breastfeeding underway. Most newborns lose 5–10 per cent of their birthweight and most take two weeks to regain it, which can be worrying.

Ask yourself: is my baby happy and contented after a feed? Is she producing lots of wet nappies? Can I hear her swallowing milk during a feed? Can I feel a change in my breasts after a feed? Does she wake and cry for feeds? If you can answer yes to these sorts of questions, your baby is feeding well. If you are not sure, then talk to your midwife, health visitor or a breastfeeding counsellor.

ASK THE EXPERT
DAPHNE METLAND
BABYCENTRE EDITOR-IN-CHIEF

My nipples are so cracked and sore from breastfeeding my newborn. What can I do?

Some experts say the best treatment for sore nipples is expressing a little colostrum or breast milk and rubbing it on your nipples. There is no evidence that using cling film or petroleum jelly is helpful. For cracked nipples, many midwives recommend a purified lanolin cream formulated especially for breastfeeding women to encourage 'moist wound healing'. Unlike petroleum jelly it allows the skin to breathe. But most important is working out why your nipples are sore. Usually it's to do with the way your baby is positioned at the breast, so seek advice from your midwife.

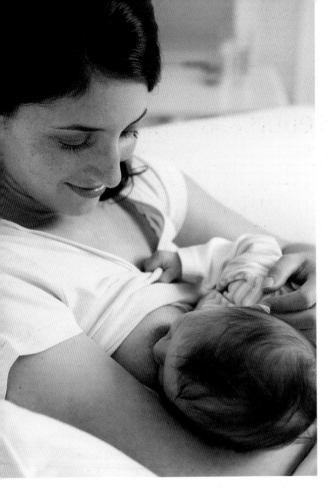

What if I encounter problems?

Some women adjust to breastfeeding easily, but others find it hard, so if you find yourself feeling discouraged, remember that you're not the only one. If you feel like giving up (or just want professional advice), consider contacting a breastfeeding counsellor (see p 226). Also, talk to your doctor, midwife or health visitor about any health concerns that may get in the way of successful breastfeeding. Breastfeeding takes practice. Give yourself as much time as you need to get it down to a fine art. If for some reason you are unable to breastfeed, you should give yourself a pat on the back for at least trying. There is much more to good parenting than breastfeeding alone.

THE BENEFITS Breastfeeding is convenient, with nothing to wash, sterilize or prepare. Once it's going well, you'll probably find you enjoy it and feel a real sense of achievement to see your baby growing and developing – and it's all your own work.

Is what I eat and drink likely to affect my breast milk?

Substances such as caffeine, alcohol and other toxins can pass from your blood into your breast milk, so excessive amounts should be avoided. Nicotine from cigarettes and drugs also pass into your breast milk and should be avoided (your doctor can advise you on the safety of taking prescribed medications).

You'll be able to work out if your baby is sensitive to something you eat or drink, because she'll show her discomfort by being unsettled after feeds, crying inconsolably or sleeping badly. Some women find that hot or spicy foods upset their babies, but food-induced irritability differs markedly from one baby to the next – trial and error may be your best guide. If you find you can eat certain foods without making your baby unhappy, then dig in.

JUST THE FACTS
WHY BREAST IS BEST

Breastfeeding exclusively for six months is recommended for the following reasons:

- *Breast milk is a complete food source; it contains all the nutrients your baby needs – at least 400 of them – including hormones and disease-fighting compounds that are not found in formula milk.*

- *The nutritional make-up of breast milk adjusts to your baby's needs as she grows and develops.*

- *Breastfeeding exclusively for at least three months may help to prevent respiratory illness in babies. If you breastfeed for at least four months, you may lower your baby's risk of catching ear infections.*

- *When you breastfeed, your baby thrives on the skin-to-skin contact and being held close. You will, too.*

How do I bottlefeed my baby?

The most important aspects of bottlefeeding are being rigorous about sterilizing the equipment and ensuring you make up the formula accurately. It's still possible to enjoy intimacy with your baby by giving him a bottle and it means that your partner can take an equal share in the feeding and they can enjoy time together.

How often should I bottlefeed my baby?

Most experts agree that you shouldn't follow a rigid schedule in the early weeks, though you may be able to work out an approximate pattern within a month or two. Offer the bottle every two to three hours at first, or when your baby seems hungry. Don't force more than he seems ready to eat.

How do I make up formula milk?

Follow the instructions on the packet carefully and use cooled boiled water. Fill the bottle to the marked level. It's important to put the water in the bottle first, not the powder, as this way the ratio of water to powder is correct. Measure the milk powder with the scoop provided, use the back of a knife to level off the scoop, and avoid packing the powder down. Add this to the water in the bottle. Put the teat and cover on, and then shake well. Don't be tempted to add extra scoops of formula powder as this can make your baby ill. You may find it easier to make up enough feed for the whole day at once. You can store bottles in the fridge for up to 24 hours. You can also buy pre-measured powder or long-life pre-mixed milk, which is more convenient, but tends to cost more.

Do I need to sterilize the bottles?

Yes, before you first use new bottles and teats, and each time that you use them, they need to be washed and sterilized carefully. You will need a steam sterilizer, or a microwave sterilizer, or you can use sterilizing solution. You can also sterilize by boiling the bottles and teats for at least 10 minutes. You should sterilize bottlefeeding equipment for at least your baby's first year. An infant's immune system is still immature and susceptible to infection between 6 and 12 months and the bugs that stick to milk curds in partially cleansed bottles can be particularly nasty. By the time your baby is a year old, he has started to produce his own antibodies and is more resistant to harmful germs.

What's the best way to warm a bottle?

Warm a bottle in a pan, jug or bowl of hot – not boiling – water. You can also buy a bottle warmer specially designed for this purpose. It's best not to use a microwave because it heats unevenly and can create hot pockets, leading to burns. The process may also break down vital nutrients.

QUICK TIP

Try to roughly gauge how much formula your baby will be taking per feed, so that there aren't vast amounts left over each time. Remember you can always make up more if necessary. If you have made bottles up and stored them in the fridge, they need to be discarded after 24 hours.

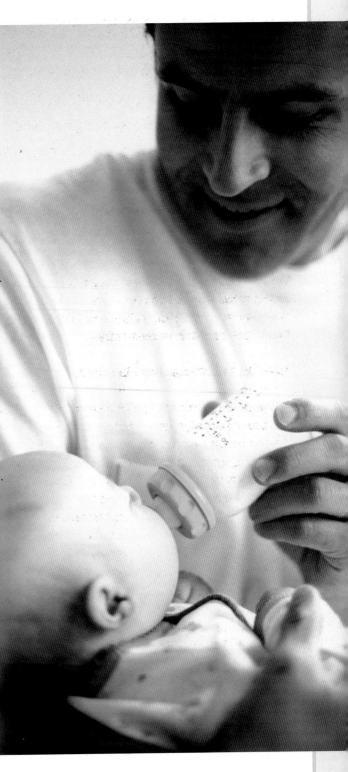

How can I make sure my baby is drinking from his bottle comfortably?

Like so much with babies, you'll need to listen and observe. If you hear a lot of noisy sucking sounds while he drinks, he may be taking in too much air. To help your baby swallow less air, hold him at a 45-degree angle. Also take care to tilt the bottle so that the teat and neck are always filled with formula. *Never* leave your baby to feed unattended by propping up the bottle – he could choke.

If my baby hasn't quite finished his bottle can I give him the rest later?

It's not advisable to keep formula milk out of the fridge for longer than an hour. If your baby doesn't finish all his milk, throw it away. He has naturally occurring bacteria in his saliva that can pass through the teat into the formula and bacteria thrive in warm, milky environments. This advice also applies to expressed breastmilk and baby foods.

How do I know if my baby is getting enough formula?

As a rough guide, babies who haven't started solids need around 71–76.7 ml (2.5–2.7 oz) of formula for each 453 g (1 lb) of body weight every 24 hours. Therefore, a 4.52 kg (10 lb) baby needs about 710–767 ml (25–27 oz) in a day. This is only a general rule of thumb. Just as your appetite varies with each meal, your baby isn't going to take the same amount each time. Don't force your baby to finish a bottle, even if there is only a little bit left. And keep a track of his nappies: at least six a day should be soaked with clear to pale yellow urine.

DAD TIME *Bottlefeeding formula milk or expressed breast milk will give your partner an additional opportunity to be involved in the care of his baby, and help with bonding. It will also give you a well-earned rest.*

What can I do to help my baby to settle?

Babies don't understand the difference between night and day for some time so you can expect to have your sleep disturbed for the first few months. The best way you can help your baby is by teaching her to fall asleep on her own; that way she is less dependent on you to help her to settle or fall back to sleep when she wakes at night.

Should I try to leave my baby to fall asleep on her own?

When she's 6–8 weeks old, you could start giving your baby a chance to fall asleep on her own. The best way to do this is to put her down when she's sleepy but still awake. If you rock your baby to sleep every night for the first few weeks, she will expect the same later on. If you leave her alone to sleep, she will learn to expect that, too. This is why some experts advise against rocking or breastfeeding a baby to sleep, even at this young age. To establish a predictable pattern, you need to adopt the same strategy every night.

Should I go to my baby when she cries?

You could try waiting a few minutes to see if she's really upset and awake, and then go in, reassure and comfort her without taking her out of the cot. Instead, pat and soothe her with your hand and talk to her. It's also a good idea to develop a calm bedtime routine, which can involve a story and bath. If you follow a set pattern every night, your baby will quickly come to appreciate the consistency.

What is 'swaddling' and how do I do it?

Swaddling is an age-old technique for making a baby feel secure. Although it's fallen out of favour in the Western world, many other cultures still use it. To swaddle your baby, spread a cotton cot sheet out flat, with one corner folded over a little. Lay your baby face up on the sheet with her neck resting against the fold. Wrap the left corner of the sheet over her body and tuck it in beneath her. Bring the bottom corner over her feet, and then wrap the right corner around her, leaving only her head and neck exposed. Don't cover your baby's

JUST THE FACTS
SAFE SLEEPING

The Foundation for the Study of Infant Deaths (see p 227) recommends that babies sleep in a cot next to their parents' bed for the first six months. Also:

- *Put your baby down on her back to sleep, not her front or her side.*
- *Make sure her feet are at the end of the cot so she can't wriggle down under the blankets.*
- *Try to keep your baby's room at a temperature of around 18°C (64° F). On very hot nights, dress her in just a vest and nappy.*
- *For bedding, use a sheet and cellular blankets.*
- *Check that your baby isn't getting too hot or too cold by feeling her stomach. Don't judge her temperature by feeling her hands or feet.*
- *Do not give your baby a pillow to sleep on or use cot bumpers.*
- *Sheepskins are okay for daytime naps, but not for nighttime sleeping.*

face with the sheet, since that could cause her to suffocate. Beware of overheating your baby; the aim is to make her feel secure rather than keep her warm. Avoid using a blanket for swaddling, and make sure you don't wrap your baby too tightly, or her circulation could be affected. Swaddling creates a slight pressure around your baby's body that may give her a sense of security because it mirrors the pressure she would have felt in the uterus. For some babies it becomes the trigger for sleep; others don't enjoy it. Try it and see!

Is it safe for our baby to sleep in our bed with us?

Some research suggests that co-sleeping may reduce the risk of cot death because small babies cannot control their body temperature easily. Co-sleeping allows mother and baby to act as a thermostatic unit – when the baby heats up, the mother cools down, bringing her baby's temperature down with hers. Many small babies have breathing pauses (apnoea). Co-sleeping allows you to be aware of these pauses, even in your sleep. You move or make sounds that bring your baby to a brief arousal so that she can tune into your breathing and join in again, without waking fully.

However, other studies show that the risk of cot death increases when one or both co-sleeping parents is drunk, has taken drugs, is a smoker or is obese. A study published in the medical journal *The Lancet* in 2004 also suggests that the risk of cot death increases if parents sleep with a baby who is younger than eight weeks old (regardless of whether they've been drinking, smoking or taking drugs). For this reason, the Foundation for the Study of Infant Deaths (see p 227) recommends that your baby sleeps next to you in a cot, not with you, for the first six months of life. That way your baby can sleep under her own bedding, but still be within sight and sound of you.

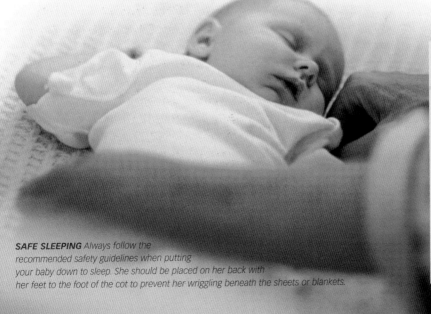

SAFE SLEEPING *Always follow the recommended safety guidelines when putting your baby down to sleep. She should be placed on her back with her feet to the foot of the cot to prevent her wriggling beneath the sheets or blankets.*

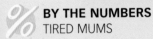

BY THE NUMBERS
TIRED MUMS

How do you cope when you need more sleep?

45% *I don't – I'm exhausted.*
39% *I sleep when my baby sleeps.*
10% *I take a nap when my partner gets home.*
4% *I leave her with a friend or a relative for a while*

Source: Based on a BabyCentre. co.uk poll of 2,597 mums.

How will I feel physically after the birth?

Childbirth puts a huge strain on your body and it's normal to experience some discomfort. Be patient and give yourself time – it may be a while before you feel back to your 'old self. At the six-week check with your doctor you will have a thorough physical examination and an opportunity to discuss any health concerns.

How sore will I be after delivering my baby vaginally?

Giving birth is an amazing and miraculous process, but it is also painful. If your baby (probably weighing upward of 2.7 kg/6 lb) has entered the world via your vagina, your perineum (the area between your vagina and back passage) will probably feel bruised and stretched afterwards. The degree of discomfort varies greatly, but it can usually be relieved by using cold packs and having a daily shower or bath.

If you had to have an episiotomy (see p 182), or a tear of the tissues around your vagina, you will also have to contend with the pain of the wound and the discomfort of the stitches in the early days. The perineum is an extremely sensitive site for a cut or stitches, and women report a wide range of pain, from mild to excruciating. Most women find that it takes 7–10 days for the wound to heal, though they may experience some pain for a month.

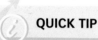

QUICK TIP

Drink plenty in the days following the birth to speed up the process of eliminating the extra water you retained through pregnancy. All the extra fluid will start seeping out in the form of sweat and urine. New mothers perspire a lot, and they often produce twice the usual amount of urine each day. Drinking also helps with breastfeeding as your body needs lots of fluid to make breast milk.

Will I experience any bleeding after I've given birth?

Every woman bleeds after having a baby, whether it's born vaginally or by Caesarean. Postnatal discharge, known as lochia, is the way your body discharges leftover blood, mucus and placental tissue from the uterus. The discharge comes from the site where the placenta was attached to the uterus and it may come out in gushes or flow more evenly. After the initial bleeding slows, and as the healing continues, the flow of lochia will turn from bright red to pink, and eventually to yellow-white.

You may bleed for as little as 2–3 weeks or as long as six weeks after birth. The flow will taper off very gradually. Red lochia should not persist for more than two weeks, although if you try to do too much too soon, it may start flowing again. If you pass bright red blood, it's a sign to slow down. Make sure you stock up on maternity towels: tampons are off limits for the first six weeks because they can introduce bacteria into your still-healing uterus and cause infection.

In rare cases, some women will have a delayed postpartum haemorrhage. If you do have abnormally heavy bleeding (saturating a sanitary pad within an hour), call your doctor or midwife immediately. This could be a sign that a piece of the placenta was left inside your uterus, that your uterus isn't shrinking properly or that you have an infection. If you're bleeding briskly and feel faint, call an ambulance.

I haven't been able to control my bladder since giving birth. Why is this?

Urinary stress incontinence is one of the least talked about side-effects of pregnancy and giving birth. If you had trouble controlling your urine during pregnancy, you're likely to have the same problem after you've had your baby. But rest assured that it is a relatively common and usually temporary postnatal problem.

Conventional wisdom holds that urinary stress incontinence happens when the pelvic floor muscles that support your bladder and urethra are too weak after childbirth to shut off the stream of urine. But new research suggests that postnatal incontinence may be the result of changes to your body during pregnancy rather than the result of damage to your perineum during childbirth.

If you had an epidural or spinal block (see p 172), you may find that your perineal nerves are so numb in the first few days after birth that you can't tell when you need to urinate. Your midwife will remind you and help you to go to the toilet soon after giving birth. Even though there is some debate over the cause of postnatal urinary stress incontinence, doing regular pelvic floor exercises (see p 147) is the best way to cope with the problem. If you didn't do pelvic floor exercises before giving birth, it can take from 6 to 12 weeks after starting them postnatally to improve your bladder control.

If you have absolutely no control over the flow of your urine and feel pain when you urinate, have cloudy urine, urine with a foul smell, or a fever, you may have a urinary tract infection. Speak to your doctor or midwife.

Why do I need a six-week check?

The postnatal check, six weeks after the birth, is to check your recovery. Your doctor will examine you to check your uterus has shrunk back to the right size and examine any wounds such as a Caesarean scar or stitches from a tear, and she may check your breasts and nipples if you are breastfeeding. Your blood pressure, weight and urine will also be checked and possibly your blood for anaemia.

The doctor will also talk to you about using contraception and give you the opportunity to ask any questions. Talk to your doctor about when it is safe to resume sexual activity. Be reassured that the majority of women find sexual intercourse uncomfortable after childbirth, but it usually improves with time. If it doesn't, go back and seek advice from your doctor.

Your baby will also have a six-week check in the baby clinic to assess his overall growth and development. As well as being weighed and measured, your baby's reflexes will be checked – for example, can he grasp a finger and hold on? The doctor will also give your baby a thorough physical examination.

JUST THE FACTS
REMEDIES FOR STITCHES AND BRUISING

Some women find their stitches painful and slow to heal; others experience less discomfort. Try the following treatments to aid healing:

- *Warm water – either a bath, shower or bidet.*
- *Cool water or cooled witch hazel or gel pads. Cold showers and ice packs are no longer recommended as they constrict the blood vessels and can delay healing.*
- *Oral analgesia, such as paracetamol.*
- *Anaesthetic gels.*
- *Herbal remedies and creams – calendula, comfrey or arnica.*
- *Sitting on a cushion or rubber ring.*
- *Pelvic floor exercises (see p 147) to increase blood flow to the area and help to speed up the healing process.*

How will I feel emotionally after the birth?

Having a baby can bring much joy, but may affect you in ways you didn't expect. It's common to feel a bit low a few days after the birth and fear that you don't actually like being a mum, but be reassured that this passes quickly for most women. Bonding can also take time for some women but is usually well established within a few weeks.

What are the baby blues?

Soon after giving birth, many women encounter what's commonly called the 'baby blues' – weepiness and moodiness, and a sense of physical and emotional anti-climax. The baby blues are often linked to hormonal changes three or four days after delivery, when pregnancy hormones dissipate and milk production kicks in. In addition, arriving home from hospital can help to increase a new mother's sense of uncertainty. The blues affect 60–80 per cent of women; many find themselves exhausted, unable to sleep, or feeling trapped or anxious. Your appetite can change (you may eat more or less), or you can feel irritable, nervous, worried about being a mother, or afraid that being a mother will never feel better than this.

How long do the baby blues last?

Few women find that their sadness persists for longer than a few days. Remember, the new sense of responsibility that comes with a baby can feel overwhelming, and the reality of what parenthood involves doesn't really hit many women until their first few days at home. The baby blues are often confused with postnatal depression (see pp 208–9) because they share common symptoms, but the baby blues are not an illness and will go away on their own. No treatment is necessary other than reassurance, support, rest and time.

What is bonding?

Bonding is the intense attachment that parents develop with their baby. It's the feeling that makes you want to shower your baby with love and affection and know you would do anything to protect her. For some parents, this feeling develops within the first few days – or even minutes – of birth. For others, it may take a little longer. In the past, researchers who studied the process

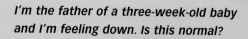

ASK THE EXPERT
ANNA MCGRAIL
BABYCENTRE EXECUTIVE EDITOR

I'm the father of a three-week-old baby and I'm feeling down. Is this normal?

Yes, it's very normal. Fathers can experience similar emotions to a new mother, and there's some evidence that new dads can become depressed after the birth of a baby as well. That's how we know that the baby blues aren't caused by hormonal changes alone. Many factors can contribute to these feelings. The most common are fear of fatherhood, financial concerns and anxieties about being a good enough dad. What often compounds the stress is that men are brought up not to share their fears. Unfortunately, keeping silent about your emotions actually increases stress. Try to talk to your partner, a friend or your doctor about anything that's worrying you. By expressing your anxieties, you're more likely to get a clearer perspective and the support you need.

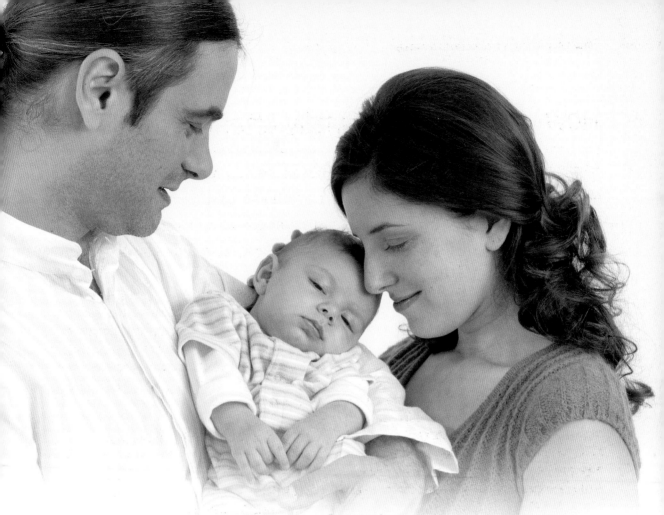

thought it was crucial to spend a lot of time with your newborn during his first few days to seal the bond right away. However, we now know that bonding can take place over time. Parents who are separated from their babies soon after delivery for medical reasons, or who adopt their children when they're weeks or months old, can also develop very close, loving relationships with their children.

What if I don't bond with my baby?

Don't worry. As long as you take care of your baby's basic needs and cuddle her, she won't suffer. Your baby is an entirely new person, one you may have to get used to before you become enmeshed. A true parent-child bond develops through everyday caring. As you get to know your baby and learn how to soothe her and enjoy her presence, your feelings will deepen. One day you'll look at your baby and

realize you're utterly filled with love for her. If, after a few weeks, you find that you don't feel more attached to and comfortable with your baby than you did on the first day, or if you actually feel detached from her or resentful of her, talk to your doctor or health visitor. Postnatal depression (see pp 208-9) is a real illness that can delay bonding, and it's best to seek help as soon as possible.

JUST FOR DAD

How you can help your partner
If your partner has the baby blues, reassure her that many women feel this way after giving birth. Just listening to her and encouraging her to cry if she wants to may be all she needs. Nurturing the nurturer is what it's all about. Help her set limits on daily activities and keep visitors to a minimum. Help her set priorities by organizing things that must be done versus things that can wait. Above all, let her know you are there for her, no matter what.

Understanding postnatal depression

When other women have got over the 'baby blues' (see p 206), a mum who has postnatal depression (PND) becomes increasingly anxious and miserable. PND is a serious medical condition that requires professional treatment, but it can be overcome with the right medical help and the support of family and friends.

When PND occurs

Some women who suffer from PND were already depressed during pregnancy. For others, the condition starts weeks or months after the birth. They have been enjoying looking after their babies but then gradually become depressed.

Signs of postnatal depression

If you suffer from several of the following symptoms for a prolonged period, seek medical advice.

- Being miserable most of the time, but especially in the mornings and/or evenings.
- Feeling that life is not worth living and you have nothing to look forward to.
- Feeling guilty and often blaming yourself.
- Being very irritable with people.
- Being tearful.
- Constantly exhausted, yet not able to sleep.
- Unable to enjoy yourself.
- Feeling that you have lost your sense of humour.
- Inability to cope; things easily get on top of you.
- Being terribly anxious about the baby, so that you're constantly seeking reassurance.
- Worried about your own health, perhaps frightened that you have some dreadful illness.
- Inability to concentrate on anything.
- Feeling that your baby is not really yours.
- Loss of sex drive.
- Low energy levels.
- Problems with memory.
- Having difficulty making decisions.

- No appetite or comfort-eating.
- Disturbed sleep, including early morning wakefulness.

'Talking' therapies

Talking about how you are feeling to someone who understands depression can be very effective. Your doctor may be able to refer you to a counsellor, or your health visitor may be trained in counselling skills. You could also contact the Association for Postnatal Illness (see p 226) who can put you in touch with a trained volunteer. Just offloading on to your partner, relative or friend may help to a degree, but they may find it difficult to fully understand what you are going through.

Effective medication

There are some good drugs for postnatal depression. Many women mistakenly believe that anti-depressant drugs are addictive, but this is not true. The main problem with anti-depressants is that many people don't take them properly. You must take your medication at the prescribed times and for about six months. It will be at least a couple of weeks before you start to feel better. Your doctor can prescribe an anti-depressant that won't affect your baby if you are breastfeeding.

YOUR BABY If you have PND, you may have difficulty coping with everyday tasks and feel unable to care for your baby effectively. You may also feel distant from your newborn and have difficulty bonding. With the right medical help, these problems can be overcome.

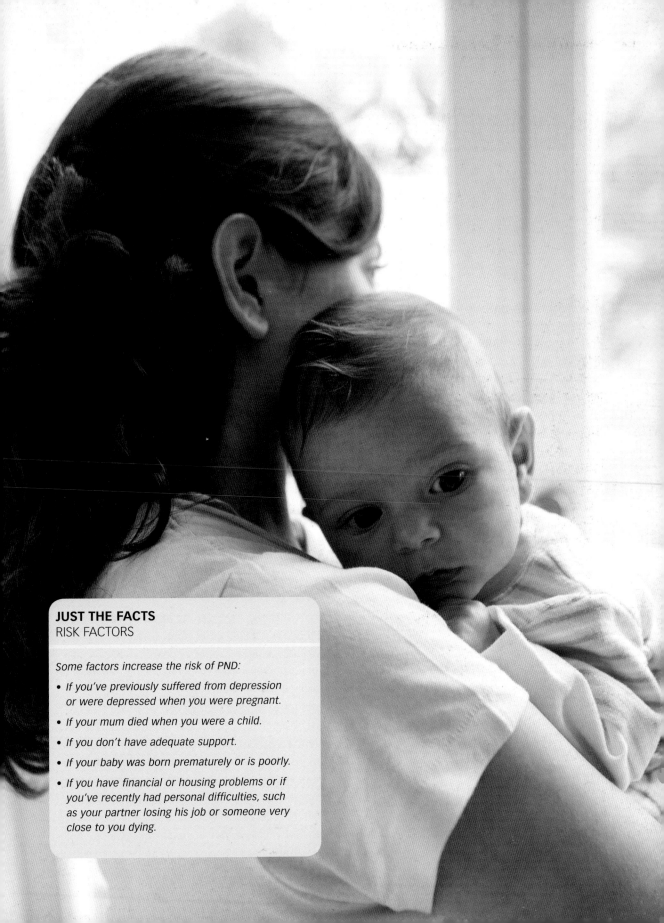

JUST THE FACTS
RISK FACTORS

Some factors increase the risk of PND:

- *If you've previously suffered from depression or were depressed when you were pregnant.*

- *If your mum died when you were a child.*

- *If you don't have adequate support.*

- *If your baby was born prematurely or is poorly.*

- *If you have financial or housing problems or if you've recently had personal difficulties, such as your partner losing his job or someone very close to you dying.*

How will I feel after having a Caesarean?

A Caesarean is a major operation so it will take a few weeks for you to make a full recovery. But with the right pain relief and support, especially once you're at home, there's no reason why you can't provide effective care for your baby. Do not, however, try to do too much too soon because that will set you back.

How will I feel emotionally after having a Caesarean?

You'll probably just be glad it's over and grateful that you – and your baby – are safely through it. You may feel elated and delighted or you may be weepy, and perhaps disappointed that you didn't manage to deliver your baby vaginally if that is what you were hoping for. If things changed very quickly during your labour and you had an emergency Caesarean, you may still feel shocked by what you have been through. It may help you to understand why a Caesarean became necessary: to do this you, and maybe your partner, need to talk to the midwife who was looking after you during labour and birth. However, try not to dwell on the birth too much; instead focus on your newborn baby.

How will I feel physically after having a Caesarean?

Even if you knew you were going to have surgery, you may still be surprised by how much it hurts afterwards. You may find you can't do anything on your own – you may need something or someone to hold on to, even to move up the bed a little. Trapped wind is another problem, especially by about day three – try tightening the abdominal muscles on an outward breath to expel the gas and drinking peppermint water, which may be available in the hospital. You'll need to use maternity pads because the bleeding from the uterus (see p 204) is the same as after a vaginal birth. Wearing knickers that are a size bigger than you really need may make the wound feel more comfortable. It will hurt to cough or laugh, but less if you support your wound with your hands.

What kind of pain relief will be available?

If you had an epidural (see pp 174–5), you may have the tube left in place for a few hours afterwards so that top-ups of painkillers can be given when you need them. If you had a general anaesthetic, you'll be offered painkilling injections in the hours and

BabyCentre Buzz

"I had a Caesarean and found it frustrating as it was painful to do lots of things. Many think it's an easy way out, but it certainly is not!" Holly

"I just want to tell worried mums that after working myself up into such a frenzy over this 'major operation' I coped very well both physically and emotionally. It was a positive experience and I have my wonderful son to show for it." Shelley

"My advice is to take all pain relief offered after the Caesarean – don't suffer in silence – and try and move about as soon as you can. Once back at home, accept all offers of help and try not to put your lower half under any strain." Ros

days after the birth. Suppositories also give effective pain relief. Don't suffer unnecessarily – if you are in pain, tell your midwife.

When will I be able to get out of bed?

At first you'll probably feel as though you'll never walk again, but as soon as six hours after the birth your midwife will probably cajole you out of bed. However hard it seems, do try to move – the earlier you can, the better for your circulation and general recovery. Once you've got out of bed the first time, next time will be easier. As well as moving around out of bed, you'll be encouraged to do ankle exercises while you're in bed, which improves circulation to your legs and helps to prevent clots.

Will I be able to breastfeed?

There's no reason at all why you shouldn't breastfeed after a Caesarean. But the pain from your scar may make things a bit more challenging in the early days, so be prepared for this and keep trying different positions until you are comfortable. Try to have someone else around when you're feeding, so you can get comfortable before you start, and then have the baby handed to you. Lying on your side may be easier than sitting up. If you do sit up to feed, tuck your baby's legs under one arm and use your other hand to guide his head towards your nipple. Make sure you move your baby to your breast, not your breast to your baby, or you'll end up with aches in your back and shoulders. Use plenty of pillows to lift your baby to the right level.

What will the scar look like?

The vast majority of Caesareans these days are performed through a horizontal incision in your bikini line. At first it will look very red and livid, but as the weeks and months go by it will gradually fade to pink. By a year or two after your operation, the scar will probably have faded to a silvery line. Although it will always be slightly lighter in colour than your normal skin it will eventually be almost invisible. Some homeopaths suggest taking arnica for several days after your delivery, to help the healing process.

I know I'll be in hospital for a few days, but how will I cope once I'm at home?

You're right that you'll stay in hospital for at least four, and probably five, days after having a Caesarean. But in some ways life will be easier once you're home – your bed, for example, will almost certainly be lower than the hospital bed and easier to get in and out of – but you can't expect to be back to normal straightaway.

It may take your body up to six months to recover after a Caesarean and many women say they don't feel completely themselves for up to a year. You'll probably be advised not to drive for five or six weeks, as turning and twisting may cause pain and having to do an emergency stop would be very painful. You shouldn't lift anything heavy including, unfortunately, a toddler if you have one, so if you have a willing helper, enlist his or her help. You can start gentle postnatal exercises (see pp 212–3) as soon as you feel ready, and this will help speed up your physical recovery.

IF YOU DO NOTHING ELSE...

- *Remember you've had major surgery so take it easy.*
- *Accept all offers of help.*
- *Experiment with different breastfeeding positions to find the one that's most comfortable for you.*
- *Keep your wound dry and ventilated.*

What can I do to get back in shape?

Like most new mothers, you may be eager to work off the extra weight you gained in pregnancy and tone your body in the weeks following the birth. Exercising can be good for you emotionally as well as physically, but be realistic about what you can achieve. You should only be aiming for gradual weight loss.

How soon can I start exercising?

Most women can do some form of exercise almost straightaway. Obstetric physiotherapists recommend starting pelvic floor exercises (see p 147) and lower tummy muscle exercises as soon after delivery as possible to help your body heal. Walking is one of the best ways to begin gentle aerobic exercise and has the added benefit that

you can do it with your baby. Many health professionals recommend that you wait until after your six-week postnatal check (see p 205) before starting exercise classes or aerobic exercises. This is mainly to allow your pelvic floor and tummy muscles to recover, and to avoid excessive bleeding (see p 204). Too much physical activity during the first few weeks after delivery can cause your vaginal flow, called lochia, to become pink or red

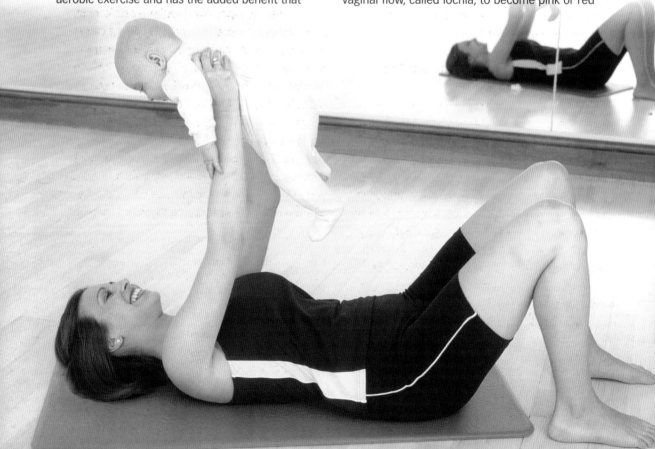

and to flow more heavily – a signal to slow down. Check with your doctor if vaginal bleeding or lochia restarts after you thought it had stopped.

If you exercised right up until delivery, you can probably safely do your pre-pregnancy workout – or at least light exercise such as abdominal exercises and stretching – from the start. If you stopped exercising during your pregnancy or are a newcomer to fitness, it is better to resume exercising more slowly.

If you find that you are leaking urine when you cough or sneeze, or are experiencing back or pubic pain, you should consult an obstetric physiotherapist before starting any exercise regime. Also, remember that your ligaments will still be a little more pliable than normal for about three to five months, so you will need to avoid over-stretching. Whenever you perform any kind of exercise after having a baby, always remember to tighten your pelvic floor muscles (see p 147) to avoid developing incontinence.

I've had a Caesarean. When can I start doing abdominal exercises?

You can begin to gently exercise your lower tummy muscles as soon as you feel ready. Begin with pelvic floor exercises (see p 147) – performed as you breathe out rather than as you breathe in – and then move on to pulling your belly button in and up at the same time (the lower tummy muscle exercise). When you can perform this easily and you can hold the contraction for 10 seconds (without holding your breath), you can then begin gentle sit-ups. Always bend your knees and tighten your pelvic floor and tummy as you gently lift your head and shoulders slightly off the floor. If your stomach

muscles 'dome' as you sit up, or you find this difficult or painful, it is too early for you to start doing sit-ups.

Can I exercise if I'm breastfeeding?

If you're breastfeeding, always try to exercise after feeding your baby. Your breasts won't feel uncomfortably full, and your baby will appreciate it, too. Recent research suggests that if a mother attempts to breastfeed immediately after rigorous exercise, her baby may shun the breast completely or feed less vigorously (this distaste should pass within 60 minutes). Provided the exercise is not too strenuous, this should not be a problem.

What's the best way to lose weight?

The immediate postnatal period is not a good time to start dieting, especially if you're breastfeeding. A good goal is to lose no more than 0.5 kg (1 lb) per week. When it comes to exercising, keep in mind that there is no such thing as 'spot reduction'. So although your abdomen may be the area you're trying to tone, the only way to shed the remaining weight is through aerobic exercise such as walking, jogging, swimming or cycling. Start slowly and build up gradually. Sit-ups are best done in conjunction with aerobic exercise – if you perform them alone you'll only strengthen the muscles below the fat, and you many not see much outward improvement.

IF YOU DO NOTHING ELSE...

Be patient and realistic about getting back into shape after you've given birth. Remember it took you nearly nine months of pregnancy to get to where you are, so it's not unreasonable to allow your body the same amount of time to recover its shape.

WORKING OUT It's all right to start exercising as early as you feel ready after the birth to get into shape. But start slowly and listen to your body. You may find that your baby enjoys taking part too!

How can we keep our relationship strong?

Caring for your newborn is likely to challenge your relationship with your partner in new ways, not least because your baby will be taking up most of your time and attention. Be prepared for a period of adjustment while you both get used to being parents and, most importantly, talk to each other about how you're feeling.

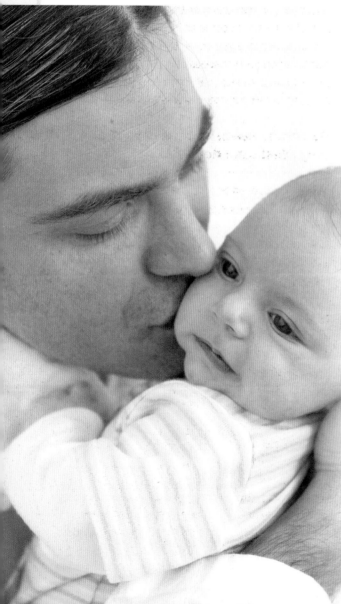

I find it hard not to interfere when my partner handles our baby. What can I do?

Try giving your partner time to perfect his newly acquired parenting skills. Many fathers who are just learning about babies and babycare are so sensitive to suggestions or criticism that they just stop doing things. You'll need to be aware of this and be willing to give up a little of your control. Of course, except for not being able to breastfeed, a dad can do everything it takes to care for a baby just as well as a mum can, especially if he gets some practice.

What's hard for some parents is that while they're practising, the baby may seem discontented. But, given time, your partner will figure out his own way of comforting his little one. If you really want your partner to be involved, leave the room or the house while the two of them work out their own relationship. Even if you're breastfeeding, you can feed your baby, hand him to dad and go out for a walk. You'll come back refreshed, and dad and baby will have had a chance to bond.

How can I get my partner to do more around the house and with our baby?

Now that you have a baby, it's important for you and your partner to talk about the changes you're going through, and how to make your new roles as parents work. Mums often complain that their partners don't 'help'. However, if you do this it implies that you have defined the work of childrearing and housework as your role and anything your partner does is 'helping' with that. But 'helping' is not really the same as sharing responsibility. Did you divide housework evenly, or did each of you 'own' certain tasks before your baby arrived? Was one person's work seen as more demanding, important or lucrative than the other's? Did this affect how you shared household tasks? Did one person take care of the other more? It really helps to think about these questions rather than taking things for granted. Try talking together about the demands of your new life, how you can divide responsibilities, and which tasks your partner could take responsibility for in the care of your baby, such as bathtime or bedtime. As any veteran parent will tell you, this is just the beginning of a new life. If you can keep the lines of communication open and figure out ways to work together as a team, your lives will become more manageable as the months go by.

How can we find time for each other?

The early months of parenthood are probably making you feel as though you never have enough time to do anything. This is very common. Even so, try as hard as you can to make time to talk to your partner regularly and schedule 'dates'. Some couples take an evening walk together while the baby sleeps in a buggy or sling. Others manage to get a babysitter so they can go out alone.

When can we have sex again?

Whenever you and your partner both feel that it's the right time for you. You may want to wait for your doctor to give you the go-ahead at your six-week postnatal check (see p 205), but you may like to try making love before this so that you can then discuss with your doctor any problems you encounter. Lubricants can be very helpful and also help with the vaginal dryness many women experience at this time. Some couples do resume their sex life within the first month, and many more resume it between one and three months, but there is a sizeable minority who wait till about the six-month mark, or even a year. There is no norm that you have to aim for.

If your partner wants sex and you don't, he might well feel rejected. Explain the physical discomfort or anxieties that are holding you back so that it doesn't become an issue between you. Full sexual intercourse doesn't have to happen the first time you feel sensuous or aroused. It may be easier to think of just cuddling at first, and gradually get used to being touched in a sexual way again.

My partner seems to be jealous of our baby. What can I do?

Jealousy is a common problem and should be addressed as soon as possible. It could be that your partner needs more time with you and reassurance that you love him as much as the baby. It may help your partner if he develops more of a relationship with the baby. If you're breastfeeding, consider expressing your milk so that your partner can help with the feeding. Make sure he has plenty of one-to-one time with your baby too.

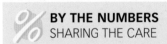

BY THE NUMBERS
SHARING THE CARE

Dads: Do you divide childcare responsibilities equally?

55% *No.*
45% *Yes.*

Source: Based on a BabyCentre.co.uk survey of 1,774 dads.

Mums: Do you divide childcare responsibilities equally?

79% *No.*
21% *Yes.*

Source: Based on a BabyCentre.co.uk survey of 2,849 mums.

Is it safe to...?

It is normal to become more concerned about your health when you become pregnant. and start to question the safety of everything you eat and drink and how you live. The guide on the following pages highlights the most common causes for concern, but if in doubt always seek advice from your midwife or doctor.

Food and drink

SAFETY METER

Almost always safe •
Usually safe •
Unknown •
May be unsafe •
Almost always unsafe •

... drink alcohol occasionally

When you drink alcohol, it reaches your developing baby via your bloodstream. Nobody really knows how light social drinking affects unborn babies and, because of this, advice varies. Some experts recommend abstaining completely. Others suggest abstaining for the first 12 weeks of pregnancy and then having only the occasional drink, while some doctors feel that having the occasional drink throughout pregnancy won't do any harm. Scientists do know that heavy drinking on a regular basis can harm a developing baby.

SAFETY METER

Almost always safe •
Usually safe •
Unknown •
May be unsafe •
Almost always unsafe •

... drink coffee

You can still enjoy coffee and other caffeinated drinks as long as you don't overdo it. Research suggests that moderate amounts of caffeine won't harm you or your baby during pregnancy. Researchers define moderate as no more than 300 mg of caffeine per day – about what you'd get in four mugs of instant coffee, six cups of tea or eight cans of cola. Any more than that is questionable. Even though no study says 300 mg or less will hurt you or your unborn baby, many women limit or cut out caffeine anyway.

SAFETY METER

Almost always safe •
Usually safe •
Unknown •
May be unsafe •
Almost always unsafe •

... drink herbal teas

All herbal preparations that are bought in the form of a 'tea bag' are considered safe for pregnancy. Although there are no food regulations that specifically address the consumption of herbal teas, any herb that is considered fine for food use is presumed to be safe for teas as well. High doses of some herbs may cause diarrhoea, vomiting and heart palpitations. If you enjoy drinking herbal teas, look on packaging labels for contents that may normally be part of your diet, such as mint or orange extracts, and steer clear of unfamiliar ingredients, such as cohosh, pennyroyal and mugwort, which are all best avoided during pregnancy.

SAFETY METER

Almost always safe •

Usually safe •

Unknown •

May be unsafe •

Almost always unsafe •

... eat barbecued food

When you're barbecuing, the biggest risk of food poisoning is from raw and undercooked meat, which is a potential source of E-coli, salmonella and campylobacter. When you are pregnant, your immune system is not functioning as well as usual, so you are more susceptible to all the bacteria responsible for food poisoning and are more likely to be affected. Although these bacteria can cause a serious illness in pregnant women, they will not cross the placenta and directly affect your baby.

SAFETY METER

Almost always safe •

Usually safe •

Unknown •

May be unsafe •

Almost always unsafe •

... eat cheese

Cheese is an important source of protein and calcium for pregnant women but certain kinds do need to be avoided. Pregnant women are advised not to eat soft, mould-ripened cheeses, such as Brie or Camembert, and blue-veined cheeses, such as Danish Blue and Stilton. This is because these cheeses are more likely to allow growth of bacteria, such as listeria, which can harm your unborn baby. However, thorough cooking should kill any listeria, so it should be safe to eat food containing soft mould-ripened or blue-veined cheeses, provided the food has been properly cooked and is piping hot all the way through. Unpasteurized cheeses imported from abroad or made by small producers are also safe to eat in pregnancy provided they are made from cow's milk and are not mould-ripened or blue-veined.

SAFETY METER

Almost always safe •

Usually safe •

Unknown •

May be unsafe •

Almost always unsafe •

... eat ready meals

Ready meals are usually safe to eat provided you follow the instructions on reheating them carefully. This is because ready meals and pre-cooked poultry may be contaminated with listeria bacteria. The germs can then multiply even at low temperatures, such as inside a supermarket chill cabinet or your fridge. Carry chilled convenience foods home in an insulated bag or box if you can. If they warm up too much during the journey, bacteria may begin to multiply. Keep the temperature inside your fridge between 0 and 4°C (32 and 39.2°F). Always use foods by their 'best before' date.

SAFETY METER

Almost always safe •

Usually safe •

Unknown •

May be unsafe •

Almost always unsafe •

... eat pâté (especially liver pâté)

If the pâté is made from liver then it should be avoided altogether during pregnancy. Experts recommend that pregnant women – and those planning to become pregnant – should not eat liver or any liver products, such as liver sausage or pâté. Liver contains very high levels of the retinol form of Vitamin A, which can be harmful to your developing baby. Other forms of pâté, including those made from vegetables or fish, should also be avoided during pregnancy to reduce the risk of listeria infection unless it is tinned or labelled UHT (ultra heat-treated).

... eat peanuts

The UK government recommends that certain women avoid eating peanuts while they are pregnant. You are advised to avoid peanuts if you, your baby's father, or one of your previous children has an allergy-related condition, such as eczema, asthma or hayfever, or if any of you have had an allergic response to, for example, strawberries, shellfish or peanuts. It is only peanuts that should be avoided by some women – other nuts, such as Brazil nuts, hazelnuts, walnuts and cashew nuts are safe.

... eat bio-yoghurts and drinks

Many women think that yoghurts that are labelled 'live' or 'bio', or that contain probiotic bacteria, are unsafe to have during pregnancy. However, this isn't true. Any type of yoghurt is safe to eat during pregnancy. Probiotic drinks, fromage frais, crème fraîche and soured cream are also safe to have. You might want to choose low-fat yoghurts rather than full-fat as they contain just as much calcium. Do keep an eye on the sugar content, though, as some are quite sugary. As an alternative to flavoured yoghurts, try plain yoghurt with a little honey or jam, instead.

... eat rare or raw meat

Raw, rare and undercooked meat or poultry of any kind is best avoided in pregnancy. It may contain the salmonella bacteria and the toxoplasmosis parasite. Store raw meat carefully so that the juice cannot drip on to other food. Do not put cooked food down on the same chopping board or surface that has been used for raw meat without thoroughly cleaning the surface first. If you are marinating meat, keep it refrigerated and in a covered dish. Wash your hands and all utensils after handling raw meat, and cook poultry and meat until no pink remains and the juices run clear. Test this by sticking a fork or skewer into the thickest part of the meat. Take special care with grilled or barbecued meat: it may appear black on the outside but remain underdone and pink on the inside.

... eat raw seafood

Some types of sushi (such as steamed crab and cooked eel) are fine to eat while you're pregnant. However, fresh, raw seafood is potentially risky because it can contain parasites such as tapeworms, which, if they grow large enough, could rob your body of nutrients needed for your growing baby. Freezing and cooking kills the parasites. Oysters and other shellfish should be avoided during pregnancy, unless they are part of a hot meal and have been thoroughly cooked. This is because, when they are raw, these types of seafood might be contaminated with harmful bacteria and viruses. These bacteria and viruses are usually killed by thorough cooking.

SAFETY METER

Almost always safe •

Usually safe •

Unknown •

May be unsafe •

Almost always unsafe •

... eat soft-boiled or raw eggs

Eating soft-boiled or raw eggs is not recommended while you are pregnant because of the small risk that the eggs may be contaminated with salmonella bacteria. Eggs that have been cooked until both the yolk and the white are solid are safe. It's best to avoid eating home-made sorbets, meringues, mousses, and mayonnaise, as raw eggs are sometimes used to make these foods. Supermarket mayonnaise sold in jars is made with pasteurized eggs, so it is safe to eat during pregnancy.

SAFETY METER

Almost always safe •

Usually safe •

Unknown •

May be unsafe •

Almost always unsafe •

... eat tuna

The Food Standards Agency (see p 227) advises that pregnant and breastfeeding women, and those who intend to become pregnant, should limit the amount of tuna they eat. You should eat no more than two medium-size cans or one fresh tuna steak per week. This advice is based on two medium-size cans with a drained weight of 140 g (5 oz) per can and a steak weighing about 140 g (5 oz) cooked or 170 g (6 oz) raw. This is comparable to six rounds of tuna sandwiches or three tuna salads per week. This advice is given because of the levels of mercury in tuna, which at high levels can harm a baby's developing nervous system. For the same reason, avoid eating shark, swordfish and marlin.

Health and medicines

SAFETY METER

Almost always safe •

Usually safe •

Unknown •

May be unsafe •

Almost always unsafe •

... take medicines for acne

Oral medications containing retinoic acid (Roaccutane) are used to treat severe acne. Roaccutane is one medicine that is definitely not safe to take during pregnancy because it's known to cause birth defects such as learning disabilities, various brain malformations, heart defects, and facial abnormalities. Experts also associate it with an increased incidence of miscarriage. Other topical treatments for acne containing tretinoin are also not recommended for use during pregnancy.

SAFETY METER

Almost always safe •

Usually safe •

Unknown •

May be unsafe •

Almost always unsafe •

... use aromatherapy oils

The relaxing and soothing effects of aromatherapy oils, especially when used with massage, can improve your well-being and general health, although there are some you shouldn't use during pregnancy. If you're pregnant, you would be wise to consult a professional aromatherapist (see p 226) to find out which you should avoid. Some practitioners recommend that a pregnant woman should not use aromatherapy oils in the first trimester, but will be happy to treat you with a careful selection of safe essential oils during the rest of your pregnancy.

SAFETY METER

Almost always safe •

Usually safe •

Unknown •

May be unsafe •

Almost always unsafe •

... use an asthma inhaler

Not only is using an asthma inhaler safe during pregnancy, its use is recommended to keep your asthma under control. Although most women with asthma have perfectly normal, healthy babies, uncontrolled asthma can result in too little oxygen getting to the baby, increasing the risk for low birthweight and other problems. Uncontrolled asthma can also increase your risk for pregnancy complications such as pre-eclampsia (see p 135) – symptoms include swelling, high blood pressure and protein in the urine – and excessive vomiting. Your doctor will know which medicines are appropriate for your particular situation. In general, doctors recommend using the minimum amount of medication necessary to maintain control of asthma symptoms during pregnancy. They also recommend using the drugs that have been around the longest because they know more about their safety. Experts recommend inhalers over pills because less of the medicine reaches your developing baby.

SAFETY METER

Almost always safe •

Usually safe •

Unknown •

May be unsafe •

Almost always unsafe •

... take evening primrose oil

In recent years, evening primrose oil has been withdrawn as a licensed medicinal product, because research has not shown enough evidence to say that it is effective. There are no safety issues with the product, but the British National Formulary (a book that lists all drugs licensed in the UK) did record it as needing to be used with caution in pregnancy. This is often advised if human research has not been carried out in pregnant women and the effects on the baby are not fully known.

SAFETY METER

Almost always safe •

Usually safe •

Unknown •

May be unsafe •

Almost always unsafe •

... have fillings at the dentist

Although there is no evidence of health risks associated with mercury amalgam fillings, they are not recommended during pregnancy. Your dentist can suggest alternatives. Make sure the dentist knows you are pregnant so that he or she can decide on the best method of treatment. During pregnancy, you are more likely to get a build-up of plaque, your gums are more likely to bleed, and there is a greater chance of them becoming inflamed or infected, which can lead to tooth decay. Make regular and thorough teeth-cleaning part of your routine.

SAFETY METER

Almost always safe •

Usually safe •

Unknown •

May be unsafe •

Almost always unsafe •

... take pregnancy fish oil supplements

There are two types of fish oil supplement – those made from the body of the fish and those made from the liver. Fish oils derived from the body of the fish contain omega-3 fatty acids. These are essential for your baby's developing eyes and brain, and there are several safe fish-oil supplements specially formulated for pregnant women. However, supplements made from the liver of the fish, such as cod liver oil, contain the retinol form of vitamin A, which could be harmful to your baby, and these should be avoided altogether in pregnancy.

... have a flu jab

The flu jab used in the UK is prepared from an inactivated virus and there is no evidence that it's harmful to unborn babies. However, as with all drugs in pregnancy, it's recommended that you don't have it unless there is a clear medical reason. If you do develop flu-like symptoms, such as fever, chills, achiness and loss of appetite, speak to your midwife or doctor. It's important to keep your temperature as normal as possible while you are pregnant, so avoid the temptation to sweat it out under a duvet.

... take Prozac

Researchers have examined the effects of Prozac (commonly used to treat depression and other problems) in more than 1,000 pregnant women and found that those women were no more likely to give birth to a baby with a major birth defect than other women. While one study did show a slightly greater risk of miscarriage among women on the drug, many others have not. If you take Prozac for depression, continuing your treatment during pregnancy may make you better able to care for yourself and your baby. But before you make the decision, discuss the risks and benefits with your doctor.

... smoke

No. Apart from smoking's well-known dangers to anyone, such as increased risk of heart disease and cancer, women who smoke during pregnancy are at greater risk of giving birth to low-birthweight babies. On average, babies born to women who smoked during pregnancy are almost half a pound lighter than those born to women who didn't smoke. Low birthweight is one of the leading causes of infant illness, disability and death. The evidence that cigarette smoking may have other harmful effects on the unborn baby is more controversial, but other possible problems associated with smoking include ectopic pregnancy and miscarriage (see p 18–19), problems with the placenta, vaginal bleeding, premature delivery and sudden infant death.

... be vaccinated

Ideally, pregnant women should avoid being vaccinated, since antibodies in the virus could harm your baby. Live vaccines are particularly risky. The best rule is to simply avoid travelling during your pregnancy to countries where vaccinations are needed. If you can't avoid going to such places (perhaps because of your work) consult your doctor to find out which vaccinations each country you're visiting requires. Some vaccines, such as that for yellow fever, pose potential risks to pregnant women; you shouldn't have these unless you can't avoid travelling to an infected area. Others, such as hepatitis B, carry a lower risk.

... have an X-ray

It depends on the type of X-ray you need and exactly how much radiation you're going to be exposed to. The greater your exposure to radiation, the greater the risk to your baby. Most diagnostic X-rays (dental X-rays, for example) do not expose your baby to high enough levels to cause a problem. Fetal exposure over ten rads (the unit of measurement for absorbed radiation) has been shown to increase the risks for learning disabilities and eye abnormalities, but it's rare for a diagnostic X-ray to exceed five rads. Although the risk from diagnostic X-rays is low, experts often recommend that women postpone getting unnecessary X-rays until after giving birth.

SAFETY METER

Almost always safe •
Usually safe •
Unknown •
May be unsafe •
Almost always unsafe •

Beauty and fashion

... colour or perm my hair

You may have heard that it is not safe to dye or perm your hair while you are pregnant, possibly from your mother or grandmother. This is because research carried out in the 1970s and 1980s showed that chemicals used in hair preparations at that time could be harmful to unborn babies. These days the chemicals used in hair dyes and perms are much less toxic and newer research has shown that they are safe for use in pregnancy. Having said that, it makes sense to limit your exposure to any chemical during pregnancy so do follow the directions on the packet carefully if dyeing your hair at home. Make sure you use gloves and dye your hair in a well ventilated room. Or, alternatively, you could switch to a vegetable dye – some are just as effective as the synthetic versions.

SAFETY METER

Almost always safe •
Usually safe •
Unknown •
May be unsafe •
Almost always unsafe •

... use a sunbed

Many pregnant women find that their skin is more sensitive and that they are much more susceptible to sunburn. If this applies to you, be liberal in your use of sunscreen and avoid the sun if possible. In pregnancy, levels of melanocyte-stimulating hormone are higher in the body, and this makes pregnant women prone to excessive skin pigmentation. If you get chloasma (see p 96), it can be a sign that your skin will react more strongly to sunlight than usual. The chloasma may be increased if you sunbathe or use a sunbed. In addition, lying in the sun for hours increases the risk of overheating and dehydration. No definitive studies have been carried out about how exposure either to sunlight or to artificial ultraviolet rays affects an unborn baby. Some studies suggest there may be a link between exposure to ultraviolet rays and folic acid deficiency because folic acid can be broken down by strong sunlight.

SAFETY METER

Almost always safe •
Usually safe •
Unknown •
May be unsafe •
Almost always unsafe •

... wear underwired bras

There does not seem to be any concrete evidence to show that wearing underwired bras during pregnancy may be harmful. However, there appears to be a potential risk. Many midwives and retail outlets advise against purchasing underwiring in pregnancy. The reasoning behind this advice appears to be that the rigid wire may interfere with the natural changes in size and shape of the breast during pregnancy. This may obstruct the increased blood flow or 'squash' the developing milk duct system, causing pain and discomfort. If you do wear an underwired bra at any time make sure that the wire does not put pressure anywhere on the breast, and don't sleep in it.

Travel

... travel in a car with an airbag

There are no definitive guidelines on the use of airbags by pregnant women, though some manufacturers advise that mums-to-be should not sit in front seats with a passenger airbag. Safety experts recommend that all car occupants (not just pregnant women) should move their seat as far back as possible and tilt it slightly backwards. This maximizes the distance between your chest and the steering wheel. Avoid leaning or reaching forward, and sit back in the seat with as little slack in the seat belt as possible. This will reduce your forward movement in a crash and allow the airbag to inflate correctly.

... fly

Yes, in your first and second trimesters, although if your pregnancy is complicated by medical problems such as spotting, diabetes, high blood pressure, or a previous early delivery check with your doctor before travelling. You may find that your second trimester – weeks 14–27 – is a perfect time to travel. Airlines are sometimes unwilling to carry women who are past their 28th week of pregnancy because of the risk of premature labour. Always check with the airline you're using before travelling.

... use insect repellent

It depends on the type you choose. Use caution with any product that contains the chemical diethyl-3-methyl benzamide (DEET), which is often found in topical mosquito repellents. A certain amount of the chemical is absorbed through the skin into your bloodstream. In large doses, it can make you seriously ill. If you're looking for a natural alternative, use something with citronella oil in it. Citronella oil is considered safe for pregnant women.

... use a seat belt

It is always safer to use a seat belt, but it is important to wear it so that it fits across your thighs and under your bump – not across the middle of it. If the seat belt is positioned across your body, pressure from it could hurt your developing baby if you were in an accident. Experts recommend that the shoulder portion of the belt sits over your collarbone, and the lap portion is positioned as low as possible on your hips and across your upper thighs. Never place the lap portion above your abdomen.

At home and at work

... change cat litter

Cat faeces can carry a parasite that causes toxoplasmosis – an infection that isn't serious for you but can pose a danger to your developing baby. Experts recommend that pregnant women should avoid emptying the cat litter tray, but that it should be cleared every day by someone else. If you have to do it yourself, always wear gloves. The odds of contracting toxoplasmosis during pregnancy are low, and if you've had it once, you can't catch it again. It's also rare for a woman to be infected for the first time during pregnancy. If you live with cats, the likelihood is even higher that you've already contracted the disease and developed an immunity to it.

... use cleaning products

Yes, but make sure you have good ventilation where you'll be working, and use gloves to avoid getting the cleaning products on your skin. Avoid cleaning the oven, though, since it's hard to get good ventilation in such a tight space. If any fumes make you feel nauseated, get someone else to do the cleaning, or, better yet, choose products that are environmentally friendlier, such as vinegar and baking soda. Never mix different chemicals, such as ammonia and bleach, as the fumes that result can be very dangerous to anyone inhaling them.

... have very hot baths

You do need to be cautious about having very hot baths while you are pregnant as there is little known about the possible effects on the blood flowing through the placenta or on the unborn baby. If the water is too hot, you could also feel faint or sick, as it could lower your blood pressure too much. A bath that is too hot is likely to affect the colour of your skin, turning it red, and you may find yourself sweating more. The same precautions should be applied to saunas and spa baths.

SAFETY METER

Almost always safe •

Usually safe •

Unknown •

May be unsafe •

Almost always unsafe •

... paint

We don't know exactly how the chemicals and solvents used in paint affect unborn babies. The simplest and safest answer is to let someone else do the painting or save it until after your baby's born. Painting exposes you to many chemicals but, because it's so difficult to measure how much of the various substances the body actually absorbs, it is difficult to know the exact risks to pregnant women. Of particular concern is lead-based paint, commonly used before the 1970s. If you scrape lead paint, you could inhale lead dust, which could be harmful to both you and the baby. Scraping or sanding any kind of paint is definitely not recommended. Leave removal of lead-based paint to professionals, who can do it while you are out of the house.

SAFETY METER

Almost always safe •

Usually safe •

Unknown •

May be unsafe •

Almost always unsafe •

... have sex

If you have had any breakthrough bleeding or spotting in early pregnancy, your midwife or doctor may advise you not to have sexual intercourse until you reach 14 weeks. In any other circumstances, there is no physical reason why you and your partner cannot make love throughout your pregnancy. During intercourse, your partner's penis cannot damage the baby in any way. In the early months, however, tiredness, nausea, breast tenderness, general stress and worry may mean that you don't feel like having sex very often. Many women report that this feeling lifts as pregnancy progresses and the discomforts ease.

SAFETY METER

Almost always safe •

Usually safe •

Unknown •

May be unsafe •

Almost always unsafe •

... use VDUs

There is no evidence that working in front of a the visual display unit (VDU) on a computer could harm your developing baby. However, if you are positioned working at a computer for long periods of time, you may experience some physical discomfort. Sitting for long periods can cause backache, so try to get up and walk around every so often. Another good idea is to vary the way you sit. Try putting your feet up on a foot rest and using a cushion or foam wedge to support the small of your back.

SAFETY METER

Almost always safe •

Usually safe •

Unknown •

May be unsafe •

Almost always unsafe •

... work with animals

To avoid the risk of infection, pregnant women should not help to lamb or milk ewes. You should also avoid contact with newborn or miscarried lambs or the afterbirth and seek medical advice for any feverish or flu-like symptoms, if you think you may be at risk. Although salmonella and E-coli infections will not directly harm your baby during pregnancy, they can leave you feeling extremely ill. Salmonella can also occur in lizards, snakes, turtles and tortoises; in birds such as parrots, canaries, finches and pigeons; and in dogs and cats. Cattle, meanwhile, can harbour harmful E-coli bacteria. If you work with these animals while pregnant, always wash your hands thoroughly.

Useful Organizations

Action on Pre-Eclampsia
www.apec.org.uk / Tel: 020 8427 4217
Support for women at risk of or affected
by pre-eclampsia.

Active Birth Centre
www.activebirthcentre.com / Tel: 020 7281 6760
Antenatal workshops and yoga-based exercise classes.

ARC – Antenatal Results and Choices
www.arc-uk.org / Tel: 020 7631 0285
For people having antenatal tests, especially those who
are told that there is a risk of an abnormality.

Aromatherapy Organisations Council
www.aromatherapy-regulation.org.uk / Tel: 0870 7743 477
Holds a database of fully registered aromatherapists.

ASBAH (Assoc for Spina Bifida and Hydrocephalus)
www.asbah.org / Tel: 01733 555 988
Advice and practical support for people with spina bifida
and hydrocephalus and their carers.

Association for Postnatal Illness
www.apni.org / Tel: 020 7386 0868
Support for mothers suffering from postnatal illness.

**Association of Chartered Physiotherapists in
Women's Health**
www.womensphysio.com
To find a physiotherapist in your area.

Association of Reflexologists
www.aor.org.uk / Tel: 0870 5673320
To find a registered reflexologist near you.

Babyloss
www.babyloss.com
Information and support online for women and
their partners who have experienced the loss of a baby.

Birth Defects Foundation
www.birthdefects.co.uk / Tel: 08700 707020
For parents whose child has a birth defect or are
concerned about having a child with a birth defect.

Birthmark Support Group
www.birthmarksupportgroup.org.uk/ Tel: 01202 257703
Aims to provide support and information to anyone
of any age who has a birthmark and their relatives.

BLISS (Baby Life Support Systems)
www.bliss.org.uk / Tel: 0870 7700 337
Offers support and information to parents and families
of special care babies.

Breastfeeding Network
www.breastfeedingnetwork.org.uk / Tel: 0870 9008787
Information on breastfeeding and one-to-one support.

British Acupuncture Council
www.acupuncture.org.uk / Tel: 020 8735 0400
Can provide a free list of registered acupuncturists.

**British Association for Counselling and
Psychotherapy**
www.bac.co.uk / Tel: 0870 443 5219
Can provide a list of registered counsellors in your area.

British Epilepsy Association
www.epilepsy.org.uk / Tel: 0808 8005050
Information and counselling on all aspects of epilepsy.

British SPD Support Group
www.spd-uk.org / Tel: 0870 770 3236
Provides information, support and advice on pelvic pain.

Childcare Link
www.childcarelink.gov.uk / Tel: 0800 096 0296
Government body providing information about childcare
and early education services.

Children's Heart Federation
www.childrens-heart-fed.org.uk / Tel: 0808 808 5000
Information about all aspects of bringing up a child with a
heart condition.

Children's Liver Disease Foundation
www.childliverdisease.org / Tel: 0121 212 3839
Cares for all families and children affected by liver disease.

Citizens Advice Bureaux (CAB)
www.nacab.org.uk
Free and confidential advice on a wide range of issues.

CLAPA (Cleft Lip and Palate Association)
www.clapa.com / Tel: 020 7431 0033
For children and families affected by cleft lip and palate.

CLIC Sargent
www.clicsargent.com / Tel: 0845 301 0031
CLIC offers care and support to children with cancer and
leukaemia and their families.

Consumers' Association
www.which.net / Tel: 020 7770 7000
Campaigns on consumer issues and tests equipment.

Contact a Family
www.cafamily.org.uk / Tel: 0808 808 3555
Information on rare syndromes and disorders.

Continence Foundation
www.continence-foundation.org.uk / Tel: 0845 345 0165
Offers advice and information to those whose lives are affected by incontinence.

Cystic Fibrosis Trust
www.cftrust.org.uk / Tel: 020 8464 7211/0623
Dedicated to caring for those living with cystic fibrosis and to finding a cure.

Daycare Trust
www.daycaretrust.org.uk / Tel: 020 7840 3350
Information about childcare. Publishes *Check Out Childcare*, a guide to choosing childcare.

Defeating Deafness
www.defeatingdeafness.org / Tel: 0808 808 2222
Advice on deafness and hearing tests for babies and young children.

Diabetes UK
www.diabetes.org.uk / Tel: 020 7424 1030
Aims to improve the lives of people who have diabetes. Publishes a leaflet entitled *Pregnancy and diabetes*.

Disabled Parents' Network
www.disabledparentsnetwork.org.uk / Tel: 0870 2410450
A national organization of disabled parents.

Doula UK
www.doula.org.uk
Doula UK is a network of doulas run voluntarily by doulas.

Down's Syndrome Association
www.dsa-uk.com / Tel: 0845 2300 372
Supports carers of people with Down's and parents contemplating pregnancy screening or diagnostic tests.

Eating Disorders Association
www.edauk.com / Tel: 0845 634 1414
Offers support and advice on eating disorders.

Eating for Pregnancy Helpline
Tel: 0845 130 3646
Advice on all aspects of nutrition and food safety in pregnancy and for women who are trying to get pregnant.

Ectopic Pregnancy Trust
www.ectopic.org / Tel: 01895 238 025
Support for those affected by ectopic pregnancy.

Erb's Palsy Group
www.erbspalsygroup.co.uk / Tel: 0247 6413 293
Information and support for sufferers and carers.

Family Planning Association
www.fpa.org.uk / Tel: 0845 310 1334
Produces a free leaflet on contraception after birth.

Fathers Direct
www.fathersdirect.com / Tel: 020 7920 9491
Information for expectant, new, solo and unmarried dads.

Food Standards Agency
www.eatwell.gov.uk / Tel: 020 7276 8000
Provides the latest information on food safety.

Foresight
www.foresight-preconception.org.uk / Tel: 01483 427 839
Offers advice on preconceptual care.

Foundation for the Study of Infant Deaths
www.sids.org.uk/fsid / Tel: 0870 787 0054
Works to reduce the risk of cot death and offers support for bereaved families.

General Osteopathic Council
www.osteopathy.org.uk / Tel: 020 7357 6655
Can provide details of registered osteopaths.

General Register Office
www.familyrecords.gov.uk / Tel: 0870 243 7788
Provides information about how to register a birth.

Gingerbread
www.gingerbread.org.uk / Tel: 0800 018 4318
Local and national support for single-parent families.

Grandparents' Federation
www.grandparents-federation.org.uk / Tel: 01279 444964
Advice, information and publications for grandparents.

Group B Strep Support
www.gbss.org.uk / Tel: 01444 416176
Provides information and support to pregnant women affected by GBS.

Herpes Viruses Association
www.herpes.org.uk / Tel: 020 7609 9061
Provides advice and information on cold sores, genital herpes, chicken pox and shingles.

Human Fertilization and Embryology Authority
www.hfea.gov.uk / Tel: 020 7377 5077
The statutory body that regulates, licenses and collects data on fertility treatments.

Hypnotherapy Association
www.thehypnotherapyassociation.co.uk
Tel: 01257 262124
Organization of psychotherapists using hypnotherapy.

Independent Midwives Association
www.independentmidwives.org.uk
Tel: 01483 821104
Provides a list of independent midwives and lobbies for the traditional role of the midwife.

Infertility Network UK
www.infertilitynetworkuk.com / Tel: 08701 188 088
Confidential service on infertility and reproductive health.

Inland Revenue Tax Credit Helpline
www.taxcredits.inlandrevenue.gov.uk / Tel: 0845 300 3900
For information about the Working Tax Credit and the Child Tax Credit.

Institute of Complementary Medicine
www.icmedicine.co.uk / Tel: 020 7237 5165
Provides information on complementary medicine and finding a registered practitioner.

La Leche League
www.laleche.org.uk / Tel: 020 7242 1278
Helpline offering advice and information on breastfeeding, plus local group meetings.

MAMA (Meet-a-Mum Association)
www.mama.co.uk / Tel: 020 8768 0123
Friendship and support for all mothers and mothers-to-be.

Maternity Alliance
www.maternityalliance.org.uk / Tel: 020 7490 7638
Expert advice and information on antenatal care, health and safety at work, maternity leave and pay.

Miscarriage Association
www.miscarriageassociation.org.uk / Tel: 01924 200799
Support and information on all aspects of pregnancy loss.

Multiple Births Foundation
www.multiplebirths.org.uk / Tel: 020 8383 3519
Provides support to multiple birth families.

National Childbirth Trust
www.nctpregnancyandbabycare.com / Tell: 0870 444 8707
Support during pregnancy and the early months.

National Childminding Association
www.ncma.org.uk / Tel: 0800 169 4486
National charity promoting registered childminding. NCMA cannot supply a contact list of childminders in your area.

National Institute of Medical Herbalists
www.nimh.org.uk / Tel: 01392 426022
Provides a list of qualified registered herbalists.

NCT Breastfeeding Helpline
www.nct-online.org / Tel: 0870 444 8708
The National Childbirth Trust has trained breastfeeding counsellors who can offer individual advice and support.

NHS Pregnancy Smoking Helpline
www.quit.org.uk / Tel: 0800 00 2200
Provides a special intensive support service for pregnant women and those planning a baby.

NICE (National Institute for Clinical Excellence)
www.nice.org.uk / Tel: 020 7067 5800
Provides national guidance on the promotion of good health and the prevention and treatment of ill health.

Obstetric Cholestasis Support and Information Line
Tel: 0121 353 0699
Provides information on obstetric cholestasis.

Real Nappy Association
www.realnappy.com / Tel: 020 8299 4519
Information and advice on all nappy-related issues.

Relate
www.relate.org.uk / Tel: 0845 456 1310
Provides relationship counselling for couples.

SANDS (Stillbirth and Neonatal Death Society)
www.uk-sands.org / Tel: 020 7436 5881
Support for bereaved parents and their families whose baby has died at or soon after birth.

Scope
www.scope.org.uk / Tel: 0808 800 3333
The disability organization in England and Wales whose focus is people with cerebral palsy.

Serene (formerly Cry-sis)
www.our-space.co.uk/serene.htm / Tel: 020 7404 5011
For advice about excessively crying, sleepless and demanding babies and young children.

Sickle Cell Society
www.sicklecellsociety.org / Tel: 020 8961 7795
Support for sufferers and their families.

Society of Homeopaths
www.homeopathy-soh.org /Tel: 0845 4506 611
Provides a register of qualified homeopaths.

Sure Start
www.surestart.gov.uk / Tel: 0870 0002 288
Government sponsored scheme of local programmes for children under four years and their families.

Steps
www.steps-charity.org.uk/ Tel: 0871 717 0044
Support for people with lower limb abnormalities.

TAMBA (Twins and Multiple Birth Association)
www.tamba.org.uk/ Tel: 0870 770 3305
Provides national and local support.

Tommy's
www.tommys.org / Tel: 0870 777 3060
Information for parents-to-be, and health professionals to help maximize the chance of having a healthy pregnancy.

Glossary of medical terms

Amniocentesis
An amniocentesis is a diagnostic test used to determine possible genetic abnormalities, usually performed between weeks 15 and 18 of pregnancy. Amniotic fluid is withdrawn from the amniotic sac by inserting a hollow needle through the abdominal wall.

Amniotic fluid
This is the clear straw-coloured liquid in the amniotic sac in which the fetus grows. It cushions the baby against pressure and knocks, allows the baby to move around and grow without restriction, helps the lungs develop, keeps the baby at a constant temperature and provides a barrier against infection.

Apgar score
The APGAR test is routinely used one minute and five minutes (and sometimes ten minutes) after the birth to assess a newborn baby's health. It assesses five basic indicators of health: activity level, pulse, grimace (response to stimulation), appearance and respiration. The baby is given a score of 0,1 or 2 on each indicator and the scores are added up to give an overall 'Apgar score' out of a possible ten.

Birth canal
The passage between the cervix and the outside world through which the baby travels on the way to being born; usually called the vagina.

Braxton Hicks contractions
The irregular 'practice' contractions of the uterus that occur throughout pregnancy, but can be felt especially towards the end of pregnancy. They can sometimes be uncomfortable and intense, but are not usually painful.

Breech position
A baby is said to be breech presentation, or in a breech position, when it is 'bottom down' rather than 'head down' in the uterus just before birth. Either the baby's bottom or feet would be born first. Around 3–4 per cent of full-term babies are positioned this way.

Caesarean
A Caesarean, or C-section, is when the baby is delivered through an incision in the mother's abdomen and uterus. It is used when a woman cannot give birth vaginally or if the baby is in distress or danger.

Cervical weakness
This is when the cervix, under pressure from the growing uterus, painlessly opens before a pregnancy has reached full term. A weak or incompetent cervix can cause miscarriage in the second trimester or premature labour in the third, but can be treated by a cervical stitch.

Cervix
The lower end or neck of the uterus that leads into the vagina, and gradually opens during labour.

Chorionic villus sampling (CVS)
This is a diagnostic test carried out in early pregnancy, usually between weeks 8 and 10. Some of the cells that line the placenta, the chorionic villi, are removed through the cervix or abdomen. The cells are tested to see whether the fetus has Down's syndrome or other genetic abnormalities. Early results may help parents decide whether to terminate a pregnancy.

Colostrum
Colostrum is the first 'milk' the breasts produce as a precursor to breast milk. It is rich in fats, protein and antibodies, which protect the baby against infection and kick-start the immune system. Most women produce colostrum a few days before and after childbirth; some women produce small amounts of it from the fifth or sixth month of pregnancy. It is gradually replaced by breastmilk over the first week or so of breastfeeding.

Crowning
During labour, when the baby's head can be seen at the opening of the vagina, it is said to 'crown'.

Ectopic pregnancy
An ectopic pregancy occurs when a fertilized egg implants outside the uterus, usually in a fallopian tube, but it can be anywhere in the abdominal cavity. There is not enough room for a baby to grow, so an ectopic must be surgically removed to prevent rupture and damage.

EDD
The due date or estimated date of delivery (EDD) is the date when a baby's birth is expected. It is set by a doctor or midwife and is usually based on the first day of a woman's last menstrual period. An ultrasound 'dating scan' may be used to give a more accurate estimate of the due date based on measurements of the baby's size.

Engagement
Engagement, also called lightening or dropping, is when the fetus descends into the pelvic cavity. In first-time mothers, this usually happens 2–4 weeks before delivery; babies of women who have already had children usually don't engage until labour begins.

Epidural
A form of pain relief for labour in which anaesthetic is injected into the dural space around the spinal cord. An epidural numbs the lower body, decreasing or eliminating

pain, and enabling the woman to save her strength for pushing. It can completely numb the lower body, however, so she may be unable to feel the contractions when it is time to push the baby out.

External cephalic version
External cephalic version (ECV) is a procedure in which a doctor, using ultrasound images as a guide, attempts to massage a breech baby into the more favourable 'head-down' position ready for birth.

Fallopian tube
There are two fallopian tubes, one each side of the uterus, that lead from the area of the ovaries into the uterine cavity. When an egg is released, the nearest fallopian tube draws it in and transports it down to the uterus.

Fetal distress
Signs of fetal distress, including a slowed heartbeat or absence of fetal movement, are watched for throughout labour. If a fetus's life is believed to be in danger, usually because of lack of oxygen, the immediate delivery of the baby is called for.

Fetal monitoring
This is the tracking of the fetus's heartbeat and the mother's uterine contractions during labour.

Forceps delivery
A delivery in which tong-like instruments (called forceps) are used to ease the baby's head through the birth canal.

Full-term
A baby is considered full-term if it is born between 38 and 42 weeks of pregnancy.

Fundal height
The distance between the top of a pregnant woman's uterus (called the fundus) to her pubic bone. It is measured to determine fetal age.

Gestational diabetes
A type of diabetes (when blood sugar levels become too high) that develops during pregnancy. It can be treated, and usually disappears after pregnancy.

Intrauterine growth retardation
The slow growth of a fetus in the uterus, possibly resulting in a low-birthweight baby.

Jaundice
Jaundice can bring a yellow tinge to a newborn's skin; it is caused by too much bilirubin in the blood. Newborn jaundice usually begins on the second or third day of life and starts disappearing when the baby is 7–10 days old. It is sometimes corrected by special light treatment but it is harmless and soon passes.

Lanugo
Downy-like, fine hair on a fetus. Lanugo can appear as early as 15 weeks of gestation, and typically begins to disappear sometime before birth.

Linea nigra
A dark line that may develop during pregnancy, running down the abdomen and the navel. It often fades after birth but doesn't always disappear entirely.

Lochia
This is the term used to refer to the vaginal discharge of mucus, blood and tissue, which may continue for up to six weeks after the birth.

Meconium
The dark, sticky substance released from a newborn's intestines into his first bowel movements. If visible in amniotic fluid prior to delivery, it can be a sign that the fetus is in distress.

Obstetrician
A doctor or surgeon who specializes in pregnancy, childbirth and the immediate postnatal period.

Oedema
Oedema means swelling. It is caused by fluid retention in the body's tissues, and is very common during pregnancy. It can also be a sign of kidney or urological problems.

Oestrogen
A hormone produced by the ovaries that plays many roles throughout the body, but is particularly influential, along with the hormone progesterone, in regulating the reproductive cycle.

Ovulation
The moment at which a mature egg is released from the ovaries into the fallopian tubes – the time around when a woman is most likely to conceive.

Oxytocin
A hormone secreted by the pituitary gland that controls uterine contractions and stimulates the flow of breast milk. Synthetic oxytocin may be used to induce labour.

Paediatrician
A doctor who specializes in treating babies and children.

Perineum
The perineum is the area between the vagina and anus. When an episiotomy is performed, the perineum is cut.

Pethidine
A pain-relieving drug, which is related to morphine and used during labour. It is usually given as an injection into the thigh. It can cause drowsiness, dizziness and nausea.

Placenta praevia

A pregnancy-related condition where the placenta is placed abnormally low in the uterus, possibly covering the cervix, usually necessitating a Caesarean.

Pre-eclampsia

A condition that a mother may develop late in pregnancy, marked by sudden oedema, high blood pressure and protein in the urine. It can lead to eclampsia, where the mother has convulsions, so antenatal care staff monitor women carefully for the warning signs.

Premature labour

Labour that begins before 37 weeks.

Presentation

This describes the position of the baby – such as feet down (breech) or head down (vertex) – inside a woman's uterus. About 96 per cent of babies present in the vertex position; some who initially present in breech position turn before delivery begins.

Progesterone

A female hormone produced in the ovaries. It works with oestrogen to regulate the reproductive cycle.

Rhesus incompatibility

A condition in which a baby inherits a blood type from his father that is different from and incompatible with his mother's. It is usually not a problem in a first pregnancy but may cause problems with subsequent ones. Blood tests usually determine if there is a problem.

Show

A 'show' or 'bloody show' is the discharge of mucus tinged with blood that results from the mucus plug dislodging from the cervix as labour approaches.

Spina bifida

A serious congenital condition that occurs when the tube housing the central nervous system fails to close completely, which may give rise to severe disabilities.

Stillbirth

If a fetus dies in the uterus before delivery, usually after the 24th week, it is called a stillbirth. The loss of a pregnancy before 24 weeks is called a miscarriage.

Tens

Tens is short for transcutaneous electrical nerve stimulation. It is a method of pain relief consisting of a pack of electrode pads placed on the back. It discharges an electrical stimulus that interferes with the passage of pain signals to the brain and may help the body to produce endorphins, its own pain-killing hormones. The pack has a hand-held control that can be used to vary the strength of the stimulus.

Toxoplasmosis

Toxoplasmosis is a parasitic infection carried by cats' faeces and uncooked meat. It may cause stillbirth or miscarriage if a woman contracts it for the first time during pregnancy. To reduce the risk of infection, pregnant women should avoid touching a cat's litter tray and always wash their hands thoroughly after handling meat.

Transducer

A transducer is a device that emits soundwaves and transmits them to a computer, resulting in an ultrasound image.

Trimester

A trimester is a period of three months. Pregnancy consists of three trimesters.

Ultrasound

In ultrasound, high-frequency sound waves are used to create a moving image, or sonogram, on a television screen. Ultrasound images can be used to diagnose infertility and other medical problems. Often carried out at various stages of pregnancy, ultrasound scans can help to identify multiple fetuses and detect anomalies.

Uterus

The uterus is the pear-shaped, hollow organ in a woman's abdomen where an embryo will implant and develop throughout pregnancy.

Vaginal birth after Caesarean

This term is used when a woman who has previously delivered a baby by Caesarean has a vaginal delivery for a subsequent baby.

Vas deferens

The vas deferens is one of two tubes through which sperm travel from the epididymis and combine with seminal fluid ready for ejaculation. A man's vasa deferentia are severed in a vasectomy.

Ventouse extraction

In a ventouse delivery, a suction cup attached to a machine is placed on the baby's head to assist the baby's passage through the birth canal.

Vernix

The vernix is a greasy, white substance that covers a fetus in the uterus. It protects the fetus' skin.

Waters

The sac or bag of 'waters' filled with amniotic fluid in which the developing baby grows. The membranes which make up the sac may occasionally rupture naturally as labour begins, but usually remain intact until the end of the first stage of labour. The membranes may also be broken by a midwife or doctor to speed up labour.

Index

Acknowledgements

· ·

Make-up artists Victoria Barnes And Roisin Donaghy

Photography shoot assistant Bonnie Lee-Richards

Location agency www.1st-Option.com

Models' clothes Supplied by Formes and H&M

Proofreader Andi Sisodia

Indexer Chris Bernstein

Picture credits

· ·

F/C – tl – Getty Images; **F/C** – tc – Getty Images; **F/C** – tr – Getty Images; **F/C** – bl – Getty Images; **F/C** – bc – Getty Images; **F/C** – br – Photolibrary.com; **p1** – Centre – Rodale Books; **p2/3** –DP spread – ALAMY; **p6** –l – Getty Images; **p9** –Full pg – Rodale Books; **p12/13** –Full pg –Science Photo Library; **p15** – tr – Getty Images; **p19** – tr – Rodale Books; **p22/23** DP spread – Rodale Books; **p24** – cr – Artwork – illustrator Mandy Miller; **p24** – bl – Science Photo Library; **p26** – cr – Artwork – illustrator Mandy Miller; **p26** – bl – Science Photo Library; **p28** – cl – Mother & Baby Picture Library; **p28** – cl –Artwork – illustrator Mandy Miller; **p30** – cl – Mother & Baby Picture Library; **p32** – bl – Mother & Baby Picture Library; **p35** – tr – Science Photo Library; **p36** – br – MEDISCAN; **p39** – Full page – ALAMY; **p41** – tr – Artwork – illustrator Mandy Miller; **p43** – tr – Getty Images; **p45** – tl – ALAMY; **p45** –tr – Getty Images; **p47** – tl – Science Photo Library; **p49** –tl – Photolibrary.com; **p49** – tc left – Getty Images; **p49** – tc right Science Photo Library; **p49** – tr – Science Photo Library; **p50** – cr – Rodale Books; **p55** – l –Rodale Books; **p57** – tl – Getty Images; **p60** – br – Bubbles Photo Library; **p62** – l – Rodale Books; **p65** – t – Getty Images; **p68** – l – Rodale Books; **p71** – r – Rodale Books; **p74/5** – DP spread – Getty Images; **p76** – bl – Oxford Scientific Films; **p80** – Centre – Mother & Baby Picture Library; **p82** – Centre – Mother & Baby Picture Library; **p84** – bl – Science Photo Library; **p87** – bl – Artwork – illustrator Mandy Miller; **p89** – t – Rodale Books; **p91** – Full page – Rodale Books; **p91** – Inset – Rodale Books; **p93** – tl – Rodale Books; **p95** – tl – Science Photo Library; **p96** –7 Centre – Mother & Baby Picture Library; **p99** – tl – Science Photo Library; **p99** – tc leftScience Photo Library; **p99** – tc right Science Photo Library; **p99** – tr – Photolibrary.com (Royalty Free image); **p100** – bl – Rodale Books; **p103** – tc – Anthony Blake Picture Library; **p105** – r – Photolibrary.com; **p109** – r – Mother & Baby Picture Library; **p110** – r – Mother & Baby Picture Library; **p115** – t – Getty Images; **p119** – tr – Bubbles Photo Library; **p121** – t – Getty Images; **p122/3** – DP spread – Rodale Books; **p124** – cr – Artwork – illustrator Mandy Miller; **p124** – bl – Science Photo Library; **p126** – cr – Artwork – illustrator Mandy Miller; **p126** – bl – Science Photo Library; **p128** – l – Mother & Baby Picture Library; **p128** – l – Artwork – illustrator Mandy Miller; **p130** – l – Mother & Baby Picture Library; **p132** – Bottom l – Mother & Baby Picture Library; **p135** – t – Mother & Baby Picture Library; **p137** – r – Rodale Books; **p138** – l – Rodale Books; **p140/1** – Centre – Mother & Baby Picture Library; **p143** – Full pg – Science Photo Library; **p144** – bl – Mother & Baby Picture Library; **p147** – t – Mother & Baby Picture Library; **p148** – bl – MEDISCAN; **p153** – t – Rodale Books; **p156** – t – Rodale Books; **p158** – Centre – Rodale Books; **p160** – cr – Rodale Books; **p163** – t – Getty Images; **p164/5** DP spread – Rodale Books; **p167** – bl – Dorling Kindersley; **p168** – bl – Corbis (Royalty Free image); **p171** – r – Rodale Books; **p173** – tl – Mother & Baby Picture Library; **p175** – Full page – Science Photo Library; **p175** – Inset – Artwork – illustrator Mandy Miller; **p177** – Bottom – Artwork – illustrator Mandy Miller; **p179** – Bottom – Artwork – illustrator Mandy Miller; **p181** – tr – Science Photo Library; **p183** – t – Artwork – illustrator Mandy Miller; **p185** – tr – Mother & Baby Picture Library; **p185** – bl – Artwork – illustrator Mandy Miller; **p186** – cr – Getty Images; **p188** – cl – Getty Images; **p191** – t – Artwork – illustrator Mandy Miller; **p193** – Bottom – Mother & Baby Picture Library; **p194/5** DP spread – Rodale Books; **p197** – t – Rodale Books; **p199** – tl – Rodale Books; **p201** – r – Mother & Baby Picture Library; **p203** – tl – Getty Images; **p207** – t – Rodale Books; **p208/9** Full page – Rodale Books; **p212** – Bottom – Mother & Baby Picture Library; **p214** – br – Rodale Books; **Back cover** – Rodale Books x 3 images